WALKING WITH ALZHEIMER'S

A Thirty-Year Journey

WALKING WITH ALZHEIMER'S

A Thirty-Year Journey

by Shelly Kruse, M.D.

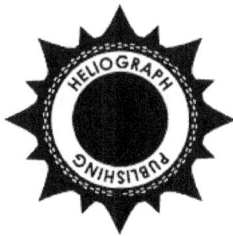

Heliograph Publishing
Clovis, California

WALKING WITH ALZHEIMER'S. Copyright © 2016 Shelly Kruse

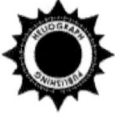

Production Assistance Provided by Heliograph Publishing
An Imprint of HBE Publishing

Layout and cover design by Joshua Muster, Heliograph Publishing

All inquiries should be addressed to:
Dr. Shelly Kruse
dr.kruse@shellykrusemd.com

Library of Congress Control Number: 0000000000

ISBN 978-1-943050-36-9 Paperback
ISBN 978-1-943050-37-6 Ebook

Printed in the United States of America
March 2016

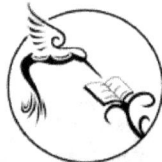

HBE PUBLISHING

Many thanks to Hazel Dixon-Cooper for her editing skills and suggestions, Judith Kammerer, librarian extrordinaire, for her speedy retrieval of medical journals.

Also, I wish to give a heart-felt thank you to every devoted nurse, aide, doctor, and staff who provided such loving care for my mother. Kerry Stutzman, RN, you were essential.

Lastly, I want to dedicate this book to my father and brother who suffered much as her caregivers, yet never wavered in their love.

TABLE OF CONTENTS

PREFACE

My mother died of Alzheimer's disease at age eighty-six. I loved her. I began to hate her. I swore I would never be like her. She had suffered from mental illness for years and was either screaming at me or crying all the time.

My eyes are the same color as hers. When I look into the mirror and stare at my reflection, my eyes look sad. I have had depression three times. Will I become her? I have so many unpleasant memories of her behavior due to her dementia, yet I miss her so much.

I am a baby boomer. We thought we could change the world. We thought we could stop the establishment, stop the war in Viet Nam, tune in, and turn off. Now, a frightening specter threatens us. As an Internist, a physician specializing in Internal Medicine, I have witnessed the puzzling incidence of early onset Alzheimer's in persons who are younger than sixty. What's happening? It's not exactly clear.

Perhaps all of those psychoactive drugs consumed during the psychedelic era have contributed to early-onset Alzheimer's in the boomer population. Maybe the DDT sprayed all over neighborhoods in the fifties and sixties is a cause. As a daughter, and as a doctor, I want answers—now.

This book is intended to be a guidebook for patients and families of Alzheimer's patients. After treating and listening to them, I have learned that they are often confused by the medical tests and X-rays their doctors order and want to know why doctors prescribe expensive medications. They also are concerned with a lack of solutions to manage difficult behaviors. My patients and their families have told me that they find that some of my colleagues rush through the exam and spend more time typing the progress note than answering their questions.

I also wrote this book to help patients understand what results they can expect from their medications, and their possible side effects. I have translated scientific language about the physiology of the disease into everyday English.

Several medical tests have been developed within the past decade which determine levels of increased risk but are not widely available. My medical training did not include anything about nutritional remedies or a role for vitamins and diet changes in the treatment and possible prevention of dementia. This book reviews many current studies regarding Alzheimer's disease prevention and treatment. This complex information is explained so that patients and families can decide whether enrolling in a clinical trial is in their interest. This book is not about selling expensive diet accessories or new drugs to make money off of desperate patients who are willing to try anything. Instead, it offers advice about the disease, recommends websites to assist with caregivers' support as well as helping patients and families find clinical trials near their home.

This book has also been an exploration for me. As the daughter of an Alzheimer's patient, I am at increased risk of the disease. The fear of getting Alzheimer's not only applies to my family, but to the families of my patients, and anyone whose family member has been diagnosed with this disease.

I want to know just how much risk I have, what kind of tests exist to find out, and whether or not I can do anything reduce my chances of getting Alzheimer's disease. And I want to share the information I have discovered as I walked with my mother through her journey with Alzheimer's disease.

My family was ravaged by this disease and we still carry the emotional scars from the ordeal. We felt so isolated, and I wish I had known we were not alone. I wrote this book to give you the information and tools to help you in your journey through this devastating disease. Please join in the fight for the cure.

CHAPTER ONE

WALKING THE GOLF COURSE

My mother, Martha Jo, developed dementia over a period of thirty years. My beloved Mom had always been a kind and gracious person. During this thirty-year journey, she raged against our family by yelling at us, throwing things, and inflicting guilt. She had developed Alzheimer's, and had attempted suicide multiple times. Every day she would tell us that she wanted to die. When it was over, all that remained for our family was guilt and the fear it would strike one of us.

I have had patients for whom this disease was not as difficult. Some remained pleasant and cooperative, and their families were able to rally around their loved one. Unfortunately, that is not the case for many others, including my mother and our family.

In 2007, at the age of eighty-two, my mother was diagnosed with Alzheimer's disease. I had gone home to visit my family in Scottsdale, Arizona from my home in California. When I entered the kitchen that morning, I observed that she could not set the table. Although she kept repeating to herself, "Four people, four coffee cups, four spoons," she walked around and around the kitchen, confused, while holding a fistful of spoons and no idea of where to place them. Although she recognized me and everyone else, I knew something was terribly wrong. My mother had set our family table three times a day for fifty years. At the time, I did not know that difficulty in completing familiar tasks was one of the ten warning signs of Alzheimer's disease

(Complete list can be downloaded from www.Alz.org).[1]

For years, Mom had suffered from anxiety and episodes of generalized shaking. Her neurologist had prescribed the long-acting anti-anxiety medicine, Klonopin, which is similar to valium. At that time, she had been on Klonopin for at least ten years.

Fortunately, my mother already had a scheduled appointment with her doctor, so I was able to accompany her and mention my observations. He ordered an electroencephalogram(EEG), a test that detects electrical activity in the brain, to determine whether or not her tremors were actually seizures.

I had to return to California the next day, and the test was done the following week. The results were normal. At her next appointment he had her complete the Mini Mental Status Exam.[2] Mom scored twenty-four points and his diagnosis was Alzheimer's disease. I was shocked. My mother's memory did not seem any worse than that of any other person her age. She knew the date and did not need help with her personal activities of daily living.

Alzheimer's? How can that be? I wondered. No one in our family had suffered from the disease. Her mother lived to be eighty-nine, and her grandfather to ninety-three. She had three uncles who each lived past eighty-five. There were no signs of dementia in any of them.

"How did she get it?" I asked him.

In 2007, her doctor couldn't give me a satisfactory answer. He did say that twenty-five percent or more of Alzheimer's patients have no other family members with the disease. I know many medical professionals who simply think people get Alzheimer's because they are old. But many elderly people don't get the disease. These responses were not good enough for me. I wanted to know. Could it be diet? Could it be her medications or exposure to pesticides?

Martha Jo had a retinal condition that affected her eyesight. Because of that and her arthritis which made getting in and out of the car difficult, she had stopped driving five years earlier. My father had taken over the shopping and bill paying. Perhaps that is why we were not aware of her condition until it was fairly advanced. Whatever it was, I wanted answers and started to look for them, for my mother's sake, the sake of my patients, and for my family. I knew my mother's health better than anyone and as I approached this mystery, I realized that I must think like the doctor I am and not the upset daughter which I also am.

In the standard practice of medicine, the first approach to a patient with a medical illness is to take a patient history. So, I did.

Martha Jo: History of the present illness—Alzheimer's disease.

My mother had led a very conventional life. She was born in Saint Louis, Missouri in the mid nineteen twenties, and graduated from college in 1947. One month later, she married my father. My brother arrived in the early fifties, and I followed four years later.

We had two cars, a new house in a suburb of Philadelphia, ate roast beef every Sunday, attended church, and prospered. Near our neighborhood were some low-lying swampy areas, and a truck would come by annually on a summer evening spraying DDT for mosquitoes. We lived in this area for eight years.

During this time, my mother had a garden in the back yard where she grew tomatoes. She loved them and would eat them every day as they ripened. I didn't like tomatoes and didn't eat them. However, my brother and I rode our bikes through the neighborhood even following the DDT truck as it made its rounds.

In 1964 we moved to a better house in Devon, Pennsylvania, which did not have DDT trucks, and our family joined the George Washington Country Club. Both my brother and mother took golf lessons and both became quite good. My mother loved the game and meeting her new golf friends. We looked like a typical middle- class family.

In 1968, our family relocated to Arizona. My father's corporate job for General Electric in King of Prussia, Pennsylvania had been eliminated when NASA cancelled GE's proposal for the Man Orbiting Lab, in favor of SKYLAB. However, a position was available for him at the GE plant in Deer Valley, Arizona.

The move to Arizona was difficult. We did not know a single person in the entire state. We had just driven three thousand miles from Devon Pennsylvania to Phoenix, and as we entered the city from the north on Interstate 17, we were greeted by a large sign that read, Phoenix City Limits—no shooting. There were several gunshot holes in the sign. This only confirmed my fears that there were still cowboys and Indians galloping along the highway on horseback. In addition, the sign was in a complete desert, with only creosote shrubs roasting in the 110 degree sun.

"This is not a good start," I smoldered to myself. "I hate this place."

I missed my friends, the deep green of our densely-forested home, and the blooming dogwoods that looked like a snow storm when we left. I stared at this terrible waste land and began to cry.

Our new house was not yet completed, and we stayed in a hotel for two weeks. My brother and I made friends at our new school, Saguaro High School, named after the tall cactus that looks like a person standing with their hands up. Dad worked long hours and made friends with the people at his office.

I did not realize how isolated my mother must have been. She had no one to talk to when we were at school and Dad was at work. Eventually, she would find her place by walking the golf course, but that was not until several years after our move to Arizona.

My mother and I had always been close. She was very loving and had nicknamed me Princess. She was a textbook fifties mom. She took pride in her life as a homemaker caring for our family. Like most teens, I had my chores, school, and friends. All of that changed one hot autumn afternoon in 1970 when I was sixteen and she forty-five.

Usually, when I got home from school, Mom and I would watch TV together. The Merv Griffin show, Password, or Hollywood Squares were our favorites.

That day, I walked in the door and said, "Hi Mom, I'm home!"

She was sitting in her chair watching TV, but instead of greeting me, she screamed, "You are such a horrible daughter!"She cursed me and called me no good.

Totally stunned, I ran to my room crying. After about an hour, I went back into the living room where Mom still sat watching the TV.

"Mom, what did I do?" I asked. "What are you so upset about?"

"Oh, Shelly, you know how much I love you," she replied, looking calm and rational. She denied being angry and said nothing had happened at all.

At first her unexplained outburst and then denial utterly confused me. But, it happened again and again. Each time she would rage at me, I would go into my room. Later, when I came out she was calm, composed, said she loved me, and denied being angry at all. I was completely baffled by her behavior. My sixteen-year-old self hadn't a clue. My brother had left for college, and at that time, my father was stressed from his job and I didn't want to add to his burden. So I kept everything to myself.

Even today I try to recall anything unusual. Had she been drinking alcohol? I don't remember seeing her drink, but it is a possibility. She was home alone all day, and Dad didn't get home until three hours after I did. However, I don't think she was drinking.

As her episodes of inexplicable anger became more frequent, I joined French Club, Girl Scouts, and American Field Service. These after-school activities assured that I would not arrive home until 5 p.m. Her attacks of rage only occurred if I were alone with her. When my father got home she acted like a devoted, contented wife and mother who served us a home-cooked dinner every night promptly at six.

In 1975, Mom resumed playing golf. Phoenix has many well-known golf courses, some of which have $200 greens' fees and another $50.00 fee for golf cart rental. However, Mom found Union Hills Golf Course, which was owned by Maricopa County. The fees were reasonable, and the club had ladies day every Tuesday morning. Mom met some other women who played weekly and joined their group. She loved golf and even won a couple of local tournaments. This was the happiest I had seen her. She looked so fit and healthy as I watched her easily lift her clubs into the car at 6 a.m. to drive out to Union Hills.

After graduating from Saguaro High School, I moved to Claremont, California to attend Pomona College. In 1982, I moved even farther away to go to medical school in Tulsa, Oklahoma, graduating in 1986.

For the remainder of her life, I kept at least four hundred miles between myself and my mother. Those angry outbursts from my mother had been like a knife in my heart, a wound from which I never recovered. When I did visit, her attacks continued, but not as often because

I rarely stayed more than three days. She always treated me as if I were sixteen, giving me chores and ordering me around.

As the decades passed, Mom developed a series of physical ailments associated with aging. She had pain in her knee, her hands, and a shoulder. As soon as one ailment resolved, two new ailments replaced it. At about the age of seventy, she stopped playing golf due to her arthritis. About the same time, she developed hypertension, and was prescribed Losartan for many years. Her blood pressure was well-controlled with this medication. Although her mind seemed to be intact, she would easily lose her temper with my father. She threw dishes at him. If he disagreed with her about anything, plates would crash onto the floor. She also became very anxious about social engagements. If friends were coming to visit, Mom would work herself into a frenzy cleaning house. Finally, my father stopped asking friends to visit because she would drive herself crazy trying to present a picture-perfect home.

Next, she decided the house was too cluttered, and started throwing away items that belonged to my father without telling him. It would take a while for him to realize these items were missing, and then she would deny knowing anything about what happened to them. In her later years, she either gave away or threw away several valuable antiques. This included an irreplaceable family heirloom, the deed to our homesteaded family farm in Illinois, which had been signed by President Andrew Jackson. We never found it.

At our family Christmas dinner in 2001, my brother asked my mother to pass the bread. She screamed at him, "What do you think I am a slave?" She slammed the bread down on the table and cursed at him. Our three faces expressed horror at her verbal attack, and dinner was immediately over. Later, my brother told me this wasn't the first time this had happened, it was just the first time it had happened in front of me. Because I lived six hundred miles away, her anger had found new targets.

At that time she was seeing five different doctors and taking six different prescriptions.

In 2002, when I arrived for my annual Christmas trip, my mother demanded I stay at a local hotel instead of my old room at home.

Mom never explained why, but I suspect she thought the house was not clean enough. When I arrived at the house, she was crying. I tried to comfort her, but she was inconsolable. After nearly thirty minutes she stopped, but could not say why she had cried. She really did not know. The next morning she wept nonstop for hours. That's when I insisted she see a psychiatrist. Although reluctant, she agreed.

The psychiatrist's diagnosis was depression. He started her on the antidepressant, Celexa, and she became much better. Her crying spells diminished and she didn't have any further temper tantrums. She still had episodes of severe anxiety and panic attacks in which she would shake all over. She also would wake up at 3 a.m. and start singing, claiming that she could not stop. About that time, I noticed her speech seemed slurred. Her gait had also changed. From a strong lady who could easily walk nine holes of golf, a distance of least one mile, her gait had become shuffling and her balance was off. She began to use a walker.

The next section on the patient history form is the diet/smoking/alcohol.

Martha Jo smoked one pack of cigarettes a week for about twenty years, and quit in 1965 when the Surgeon General report came out linking cigarettes with lung cancer and lung disease.

She consumed one to two alcoholic drinks a week with dinner. Her diet was loaded with sausages, liverwurst, hamburger, steak, and roast beef. She ate eggs and bacon at least three times a week her entire life. She did not like salad and never cooked fish. Any vegetables she ate came out of a can or were frozen.

Although by today's standards her eating habits were poor, I believe her diet was common for persons who grew up in the Midwest during the 1930's and 1940's because fresh vegetables and fruit were simply unavailable from November until June, and fresh fish was not a common item in Saint Louis. During the time we lived in Philadelphia, she would eat shellfish but never fish. I never saw her eat spinach, and she never ate blueberries. The only fresh vegetables she enjoyed were the tomatoes from her garden at our house in Springfield, Pennsylvania, the ones that had some residual DDT on them. Mom never took vitamins. Unfortunately, her eating habits were ours as well because she did all the cooking. The only difference for me was that I did not like sausage.

Depression

Today, as I review my mother's health history with the benefit of hindsight, several warning red flags appear. First, is the development of a severe depression about four years before the diagnosis of Alzheimer's, although she had a significant improvement in her symptoms from her anti-depressant.

A recent study of adults over the age of fifty who were diagnosed with a single episode of depression found that the patient's risk of eventual dementia increased by 14% when compared to adults who never had depression.[3] For patients with more than one episode of depression, their risk of eventual dementia increased 14% for each episode. A total of one thousand, two hundred thirty nine adults were followed for a median of twenty-four years. These subjects were tested every one-to-two years for depression and dementia.

Some patients who appear to be demented, may actually be depressed or even have both diagnoses. There is a great overlap of symptoms between the two such as apathy, social withdrawal, and a loss of interest in usual activities. But depression symptoms can improve with medication. This study does not address the incidence of eventual dementia for persons with depression who are younger than fifty years of age.

My father, brother, and I also agreed that Mom's angry outbursts three decades earlier were the first sign that something was wrong. With hindsight, we now can see that she had developed the tenth warning sign of Alzheimer's disease—a persistent and gradual change in mood and personality. Her anger continued to grow and her ability to control herself lessened to the point of no control at all. "The Ten Warning Signs of Alzheimer's" is at www.alz.org/alzheimers_disease_know_the_10_signs.asp.

Another red flag was her prolonged use of Klonopin. A study by Dr. S. Billioti de Gage et al. notes the correlation of long-term use of members of the valium family to the later development of dementia.[4] It is not known if this is a cause and effect—is the patient's persistent anxiety the first presenting symptom of dementia, or has the long term use of these drugs permanently damaged the memory areas of the brain? The valium group of medications all cause significant memory impairment on their own, even in younger patients. Multiple cases have been reported by the media of people taking sleeping pills which are in the valium family then driving to a fast food restaurant in the middle of the night. In the morning, they awake to find food wrappers, receipts, and even crumbs on their lips, but have no memory of leaving the house.

HOW TO DISCERN COMMON MEMORY LOSS FROM ALZHEIMER'S DISEASE

As a doctor specializing in Internal Medicine, I have had at least one hundred patients consult with me about memory loss because they were worried about developing Alzheimer's. In general, the symptoms they described were misplacing keys, phones, shoes, and personal items. These patients also noted a typical memory loss pattern, starting about age fifty, of walking into a room and forgetting the purpose of entering the room. This is a common, benign forgetfulness usually referred to as a senior moment. The usual remedy is to return to the first room, and then the memory returns of the purpose.

Anyone can misplace their keys. Usually, they are found in one of the pockets of the jacket they were wearing the last time they drove, in the car, or on the counter where items recently purchased were laid. A worrisome sign for dementia is finding keys and phones in very bizarre locations. An example is placing your cell phone in the refrigerator or leaving your keys in the shower.

Many sleepy people have placed the milk carton on the cereal shelf and the cereal in the fridge. That is just sleepiness. A diagnostic situation is having the keys in hand and not knowing how to place the key into the lock and turn it. It is benign to forget an appointment. It is another to have no recollection of ever making the appointment, or completely forgetting a conversation ever occurred.

From working with my patients, I have found that the number one presenting symptom of dementia is getting lost while driving to a familiar location, or being inside a familiar location such as a grocery store, and having no idea of where the exit or cashier is. When travelling a well-known route, a mentally normal person can sail past their destination while day dreaming or listening to the radio. Generally, in less than five minutes, they will realize they missed their turn and easily navigate back to their destination. After a few minutes, early dementia patients forget their intended goal, sail past it and keep going.

One of my patients was driving to another doctor's office about two miles from his house. He was found seventy-five miles away in a mountain town. He had just kept driving with no idea of where he was going. Driving a car is a very complex activity involving constant attention. You must be able to follow road signs, stops, and avoid collisions. As Alzheimer's begins, patients may have a series of collisions. After several of these accidents, the family may take away their keys.

The driver must also remember the streets, turns and highway exits. Behind the complex task of driving is remembering your destination. That way you can negotiate detours and take alternate routes if needed. Most adults have a map in their heads and can drive everywhere in town without relying on GPS. With Alzheimer's, that mental map is gone. The person not only forgets where they are going but how to get there. These episodes of becoming lost can be very frightening. Or, sometimes, the person just ignores it and makes poor excuses.

I have found the second most common presenting symptom of Alzheimer's can be difficulty in managing finances. The patient writes checks and does not record them. They stop balancing their checkbook each month, which results in an overdrawn account. Several of my patients have developed an inability to control their spending. They buy impulse items or expensive gifts they cannot afford to give to relatives. Despite the family telling their parent to stop buying so many unwanted gifts, he or she cannot control their spending.

Often, this loss of control is reflected in giving more than they can afford to charities. Many fall victim to scammers. The elder cannot recall how much they already spent, and sends more money. Many must have to have a relative take over their bank account, but sadly, only after thousands of dollars have been lost. Having difficulty managing finances or being victimized by a scammer is not a necessarily a sign of Alzheimer's. Some people have difficulty managing finances their entire lives. The warning sign of Alzheimer's disease is that people who had managed their finances well in the past now make large errors and don't notice.

Another sign of dementia is a new onset of loss of organization. The mail is not opened. Unpaid bills are scattered on tables in every room of the house, some of them overdue. Bills may be found in very strange locations such as the freezer. Many patients who were previously well-known for being neat and orderly become extremely disordered. The kitchen is cluttered. The once spotless house is a mess. The refrigerator may be toxic.

In 2007, after my mother's diagnosis, I always checked the refrigerator as soon as I arrived for a visit. Both of my parents had begun to eat only half of a meal. They would place the uneaten half in a wrapper and place the remainder in the refrigerator. Then, the next day they would forget to eat the remainder. I would find the dried up remains of dozens of sandwiches, half eaten soups, and rotting dinners. In 2006, my father had fallen and fractured three vertebrae in his back and was disabled himself. Although they had aide who visited daily, this person did not clean out the fridge.

Poor decision making is another symptom of early dementia as well as mental illness. They may withdraw money from a safe investment and risk it all in a get rich scheme. There can be a decline in self-control and social boundaries.

An elderly male patient of mine began to make inappropriate passes at young women. He even made passes towards nurses while sitting next to his wife. To her credit, she only rolled her eyes because she knew it was a part of his disease.

My mother was an unusual patient. Her symptoms of worsening

angry outbursts, emotional distress, and crippling anxiety overshadowed and predated her memory loss by thirty years. It is possible her symptoms were not part of dementia, but instead were the result of an undiagnosed mental illness. However, neither I nor my father and brother thought so.

What about DDT?

In 2013, researchers at Rutgers found a link between DDT exposure and Alzheimer's disease.[5] DDT was widely used from 1940 until banned in the United States in 1972. It was banned because of toxic effects on birds. Their egg shells were too thin, and broke before the young were ready to hatch. During the sixties, government agents and scientists reassured us over and over again how safe DDT was. I should have known the government was lying. But back then more people trusted the government. Now, many other toxic effects have been found.

In a research project led by Dr. Jason Richardson Phd, from Robert Wood School of Medicine, Rutgers University, blood samples of Alzheimer's patients were taken to measure dichlorodiphenyldichloroethylene (DDE), the breakdown product of DDT. Levels of DDE in the Alzheimer's group were 3.8 times higher than control patients, and the patients with the highest DDE levels were at an even higher risk. DDT and DDE are chemicals that are both stored in fat. The brain is an organ very high in cholesterol, and DDE is stored in the brain as well. Unfortunately, after exposure, nothing can rid the body of this pesticide. It appears that my conjecture was correct. Martha Jo's garden-fresh tomatoes may have been toxic with DDT. I have thought about having my DDE levels checked, but there is nothing I can do about it now. Of note, not all Alzheimer's patients had elevated DDE levels. Although banned for four decades, seventy-five percent of Americans have DDE present in their blood.

A download from the Alzheimer's Association website from April 2013, Alzheimer's Facts reports there are approximately 5.3 million people in the US who currently have Alzheimer's disease.[6] Of these, two hundred thousand are younger than age sixty-five. By 2050, that number is expected to soar to more than thirteen million as the baby boomer generation ages. The greatest incidence of Alzheimer's correlates to the patient's age. Less than 5% of patients are younger than age sixty-five. For males, aged eighty-five and above, the lifetime risk is 11%. For females in the same age group, the risk is fourteen percent.

Yet, Alzheimer's is not an inevitable part of aging. Many people survive to their first century with intact memory and brain function. So what is this strange disease? Unlike cancer, there are no survivors. It is relentless and spares none of its victims. Alzheimer's affects every race, occurs on every continent, and does not care whether you are rich or poor. But scientists have found seven factors for Alzheimer's which can reduce the risk of the disease by 50%.[7] These are a lack of exercise, obesity, diabetes mellitus, high blood pressure, smoking, low education level, and depression. A large data-based study was released at University of California in San Francisco and the San Francisco VA. The study combined the results of dozens of previous studies from 2005 to 2011. They used advanced statistics to determine the risk of each factor. They addressed the prevalence of seven risk factors of Alzheimer's disease in the adult population compared to the amount of disease in the AD population. The amount of the seven risks varied greatly between citizens of different counties. For instance, obesity in the US is 13% but worldwide is 3.4%. For the USA the study showed the highest risk factor for Alzheimer's was lack of exercise at 21%. This means Americans can lower their risk of developing AD by 21% if they exercise on a regular basis. The other six risks were depression at 15%, smoking at 11%, high blood pressure beginning in middle age at 8%, obesity at 7.3%, low education defined as not completing high school at 7%, and diabetes mellitus at 3%. Altogether this study said that it is possible for Americans to reduce their risk of developing AD by more than 50% if they reduce all seven factors. The study also reports that a 10 to 15% reduction of all seven risk factors could prevent as many as one million cases of AD world-wide and 180,000 to 490,000 cases in the US.

Risk factors do not equal causation. Obesity is a risk for AD, not a cause. Obese persons usually exercise less, and are more likely to have diabetes mellitus. They also are more likely to consume higher levels of sugar based foods and soda. They may have more medical problems such as back pain that prevents them from exercising. These would be called confounding factors. Causation is much more diffi-cult to prove. There are several additional studies in Chapter 9 about these risk factors.

In the past ten years scientists have discovered quite a lot about the physiology of the disease, and there are several FDA (Feder-al Drug Administration) approved treatments. But there is no cure. Until recent discoveries, scientists had no clue about where to at-tack the disease. But now scientists can target the disease process before symptoms appear. Now there is one possible treatment, and one hopeful vaccine. The Alzheimer's Association has a stated goal of finding a treatment that slows the disease and treats it by 2025. I hope this comes true.

CHAPTER TWO

Walking into the Doctor's Office

In thirty years of my internal medicine practice, of all the hundreds of patients who made an appointment concerned about their memory, only one patient actually did have significant memory loss.

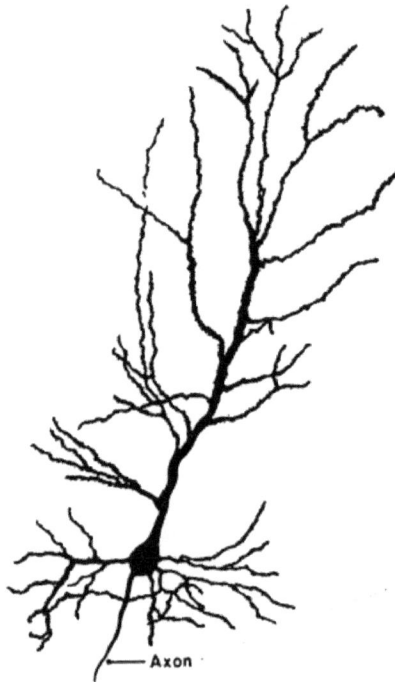

— Axon

Pyramidal cell of
cerebral cortex

Usually dementia patients refuse to believe there is anything wrong with them; their anxious spouses and family members make the appointment and accompanied their family member to their appointment. The inability to admit to having memory impairment is called denial. This is often common with mental illness as well.

These patients' response to their appointments and family concerns was varied, some would accept the diagnosis, others believed their family conspired against them and were trying to take away their money or house. Even when confronted with direct evidence of their memory loss, they denied it and made excuses such as they just weren't paying attention. They would say that everyone makes minor mistakes from time to time and their memory impairment was minimal. Many dementia patients did not believe the doctor's diagnosis either.

ORGANIC VERSUS FUNCTIONAL DEMENTIA

Dementia is an organic loss of intellectual function. Organic means there are physical findings present in the brain of affected people. This is the opposite to a functional loss of memory, in which the structures appear normal. A functional memory loss would include amnesia for an emotionally-charged event. Another functional memory loss is a blackout caused by alcohol. The alcohol prevents the memory cells from working, but the cells are normal when the toxic alcohol is not present.

DISCOVERING ALZHEIMER'S DISEASE

Alois Alzheimer, a German psychiatrist working in Frankfurt, had a patient aged fifty-one, who had short-term memory loss.[8] In 1906, after the patient died, he sent her preserved brain to Munich. Sections of her brain were sliced very thin to view under a microscope, and stained to reveal the pattern of nerve cells. Dr. Alzheimer discovered several major differences from normal adult brains.

Neurons are cells that can transmit an electrochemical impulse. There are neurons in the central nervous system: the brain and spinal cord. Other neurons travel from the spinal cord to the limbs, skin, and entire body called the peripheral nervous system. When studying this patient's brain tissue, Dr. Alzheimer's saw white patches outside of the neurons, and named these substances amyloid plaques. Some of the neurons showed structures he had never seen before. There were clumps of linear material inside the neurons which he named neuro-fibrillary tangles. Additional knowledge from the anatomy of the brains of patients with Alzheimer's disease shows that the number of neurons is significantly reduced in the areas of the brain where memory is encoded, the hippocampus.

In 1906, Dr. Alzheimer gave a lecture to his colleagues in Germany addressing his findings. He presented slides of the abnormal brain tissue and discussed the patient's memory loss. At that time, the disease was called pre-senile dementia. A decade later, the name was changed in honor of Dr. Alzheimer.

Leading theories about Alzheimer's

For decades, research has focused on the nature of the amyloid plaques. Amyloid is a general term for many types of protein collections. The word amyloid means it resembles starch under a microscope, but the amyloid plaques found in the brain are not starch. The amyloid in the brain is a normal protein present in the brains of healthy people. Although Alzheimer's patients do not seem to make more amyloid than unaffected people, they may make it in an abnormal structural form.

Precursor amyloid is a large protein, half inside the neuron cell and half outside the cell. Its function is not yet known. It is broken into pieces by enzymes, digestive chemicals that break down and recycle proteins. In Alzheimer's disease, the amyloid is broken down in the wrong place. The abnormal remnants stick together outside the cells, and seem to be toxic to the neurons. This material gets between cells and prevents the cells from communicating with each other. The sticky amyloid globs together and is not removed by the natural process of cell recycling.

This toxic material is called beta-amyloid 1-42. Scientific journals often abbreviate it as AB-42. Certain genes have been identified as creating the enzymes that cut the precursor amyloid in the wrong location. These genes are called presenilin 1 and presenilin 2. Persons with these mutations are at high risk of dementia, especially early-onset disease, before the age of sixty-five. However, only about five percent of Alzheimer's patients have one of these two mutations.

Another theory about the development of Alzheimer's disease suggests an abnormality of a long protein called tau. Just as a building has long metal girders or wooden beams that support the entire structure, neurons contain microtubules which run the length of the long axon, forming the internal framework of the neuron. In Alzheimer's disease, these tau proteins are changed by the addition of small chemical phosphorus groups. This causes the healthy tubules to lose their structure. Instead of being straight, they become tangled into a ball. Eventually, the microtubules break down and form neuro-fibrillary tangles which are located inside the neurons. A nerve with a neuro-fibrillary tangle can no longer function correctly and will die soon. Dr. Alzheimer's saw these structures with his microscope. It is possible to tap fluid from around the spinal cord and test it for the abnormal tau protein breakdown products. Having low amounts of the toxic beta-amyloid 1-42 and high amounts of the abnormal phosphorylated tau in the spinal fluid is 85% accurate in diagnosing Alzheimer's. However, this test is usually only performed at research centers, is uncomfortable, and can have rare but severe complications.

There is also a type of lipid in the blood named apo lipoprotein E ε4 (APOE ε4) associated with the development of dementia. The function of this protein is also not certain. There are six versions of this gene. Four versions of the gene are good, with a low probability of developing Alzheimer's, one version is medium, and one is clearly defective and associated with higher probability of developing the amyloid plaques. These genetic factors are not entirely understood, and those with the abnormal genes are not one hundred percent fated to develop the disease. Undoubtedly, there are more genes yet to be found.

My mother was not tested for any of these mutations. That is because most of the bearers of these mutations have early-onset disease and it is not recommended to do expensive genetic testing for patients with classic onset after age seventy-five.

OTHER COMMON TYPES OF DEMENTIA

Although Alzheimer's disease is the most common and well-known cause of dementia, there are several other diseases which are similar, affect memory, and are also progressive and non-treatable.

The second most common cause of memory loss is multi-infarct dementia or vascular dementia. These patients have had multiple small strokes. Each small stroke damages additional brain tissue. Many of these patients have very high blood pressure and a history of transient strokes which cause symptoms such as weakness in one hand, drooping of one side of the face, or slurred speech that lasts a day or two, and then resolves.

A third cause, which has been in the news frequently during the past several years, is dementia caused by multiple brain traumas. Boxers, football players, and soccer players may have repetitive brain injury. Decades after their professional careers ended, these athletes are encountering dementia at a younger age. It seems each blow to the head damages nerve cells. With time, they may recover but in some players the damage accumulates over decades and the cells die. Today's sports world has realized that even a mild concussion takes weeks, not a day or two, to resolve.

Additional causes of dementia similar to Alzheimer's disease are self-inflicted. Long-term use of methamphetamine, cocaine, nicotine, and marijuana can cause diffuse brain damage, and present in a similar manner to early onset dementia. The main difference between these is that with abstinence, drug-induced dementia does not progress.

Another mystery reveals that some autopsies of the brains of normally-functioning people who have died from other causes found the classic disease defining amyloid plaques and neuro-fibrillary tangles and yet, these people showed no evidence of Alzheimer's. In fact, it is now known that the classic changes in the brains of Alzheimer's disease can exist for one to two decades before memory impairment is noticed.

Overall brain health is certainly a factor of dementia. The brains of people with the poorest health and accumulated damage from diabetes, hypertension, and trauma are at greatest risk. We do know that what works best for heart health, such as regular exercise, healthy diet, and adequate rest is also good for brain health.

SHOULD YOU GET TESTED?

Certainly, the relatives of a person diagnosed with early onset disease should consider being tested. However, there is a large caveat about testing.

First, most people are surprised to discover there is no specific test for Alzheimer's disease. In fact, most tests are administered to rule out other causes of memory loss. In the past, we thought that the only one hundred percent accurate test was a brain biopsy. However, this is extremely risky, and we've now discovered that patients can have amyloid plaques without symptoms of dementia.

Second, if the test is ordered by a physician such as your primary care physician or a neurologist, this information will become part of your medical record.

Should you test positive and decide to purchase a long-term medical care policy, the insurance company, as part of its standard procedure, will require a written release to review your medical records. If it finds the positive test, the application will be denied. When filling out the application, if you omit information about the test, and the insurance company later discovers the test results, your omission could be considered to be fraud, and as a result, the policy would be cancelled.

An alternative suggestion for the children of Alzheimer's patients is to enroll in a prevention trial sponsored by the National Institute of Health. These test results will not appear in the medical record of the primary care physician, and test results of research patients are presumably safe from insurance company inquiries. The National Institute of Health website NIH.gov, has more information. Current treatments for prevention and treatment of Alzheimer's disease are discussed in Chapter Nine.

KEEP LEARNING

For decades, it has been a common belief that for each year of education a person seems to delay the onset of the disease by a year. Learning seems to create more connections between neurons. People with high levels of education do not have any more neurons than people who are uneducated, but it seems that as affected cells die, the increased connections allow the brain to circuit around the missing cells.

However, a more recent study shows that the link between education and dementia is not so straightforward. One of the confounding problems is that illiterate persons also have a higher risk of malnutrition.[9] Furthermore, poorly educated people begin working at an early age in low-paying jobs, work at hard labor, and may have poorer health and lack of access to health care for chronic illness such as hypertension and diabetes mellitus. High education levels are also associated with higher income and better health and nutrition.

During the office visit examination for Alzheimer's, the physician will ask many questions, and you or another family member should accompany the patient. Be sure to bring a list of all of his or her current prescription medications, including any over-the-counter vitamins, supplements, allergy medications, stomach meds and pain medication such as Tylenol or Advil. The doctor will usually administer a test called the Mini-Mental Status Exam which takes about ten minutes. Normal scores range between twenty-seven and thirty points. Mildly-impaired patients score between twenty-four to twenty-six points and patients with moderate impairment score twenty-three to eighteen points. My mother, Martha Jo, scored twenty-four on her first exam.

Patients must be able to read the questions and write their responses, as well as follow verbal instructions. The test is available in several languages. However, the administer must be able to speak clearly to the patient and understand the response. One of my patients scored an extremely low five points. However, this patient was not demented; she was illiterate and spoke only Arabic. As it turned out, her family member had difficulty translating the exam so that the patient did not understand what she was supposed to do.

Your doctor should also conduct a basic neurological exam, which consists of checking limb movement, reflexes in the arms and legs, and having the patient walk a straight line. He or she is looking for clues for dysfunction of the nervous system. For example, Parkinson's disease causes a tremor when the hands are at rest and a shudder-jerk of the biceps muscle when the elbow is bent and straightened. If dementia is suspected, most doctors will refer patients to a neurologist for more extensive testing.

In many rural counties there are no neurologists, and patients may not have the ability or means to travel to a large city. In some cities there can be a wait as long as six months to be seen by a neurologist. Likewise when an elderly patient exhibits classic and advanced symptoms, the neurologist may not be able to provide any additional services beyond the standard medicines available to the primary care physician.

Some health maintenance organizations (HMO) may limit access to specialists, leaving that decision to the primary care physician, who may face consequences about the number of referrals they generate.

Once you are referred to a specialist, he or she may conduct additional verbal and written tests as well as tests to assess short-term and long-term memory function. Short-term memory is memory for events that occurred within the last twenty-four hours. For dementia patients, memories from the distant past are intact, but they do not remember current events such as today's date and activities. Many Alzheimer's patients cannot recall what they ate ten minutes ago, but they can easily recall their childhood and life in high school.

EVERY PATIENT SHOULD ALSO HAVE THE FOLLOWING BLOOD WORK DONE.

Thyroid—People who do not make enough thyroid hormone can become mentally and physically sluggish, confused, and disoriented, which can appear identical to dementia. After being on thyroid hormone replacement their symptoms may all resolve with a month or two.

Vitamin B12, B1, and niacin—Low levels of these vitamins can cause severe neurological symptoms.

Vitamin D—Low levels of vitamin D are linked to several degenerative diseases and bone thinning. One study links low vitamin D levels with dementia, which is discussed in the following chapter.

Don't be upset if the physician asks if there is a history of alcohol abuse and/or orders a liver function test. Liver disease, either from alcohol abuse or hepatitis, can cause an encephalopathy, a brain dysfunction. Kidney failure can present in a similar fashion.

High calcium levels from overactive parathyroid glands and an excess of the hormone cortisol from the adrenal glands can all affect brain function, causing confusion and poor mental performance.

ADDITIONAL TESTS FOR DEMENTIA

An interesting test is to have the patient draw a clock and set the hands at a certain time. The results can illustrate how the ability to comprehend spatial relationship between items is affected by the disease.[10]

Most doctors will order a MRI (magnetic resonance imaging) of the brain of patients newly diagnosed with dementia. Brain tumors are unlikely. The doctor is looking for two other conditions which can cause memory impairment. The first is normal-pressure hydrocephaly in which there is a buildup of spinal cerebral fluid inside the chambers of the brain. The excess fluid compresses the brain. Treatment for this condition involves placing a drain inside the brain to remove the excess fluid. The person's brain may return to normal.

The second condition is a subdural hematoma. This is a localized collection of blood between the skull and brain. This may occur from a fall or injury which causes a slow blood leak. The cranium (skull) is hard and does not expand. Instead, the soft brain compresses. This is similar to squeezing a wet sponge. The sticky hematoma must be removed by surgery, which then allows the brain to slowly expand back to its original size.

Not every patient with dementia receives an MRI. Again, many rural counties do not have the scanning equipment. This test can cost several thousand dollars, and patients without insurance usually cannot afford it. The patient must be able to lie still for twenty minutes. Some people find the scanner to be very claustrophobic and can't tolerate being inside long enough to complete the test. Additionally, people with pacemakers, metal implants such as a hip replacement, or shrapnel wounds cannot have a MRI because of the metal in their bodies.

Another test for the study and diagnosis of Alzheimer's that is gaining popularity is the PET (Positron Emissions Tomography) scan. An MRI shows the physical features of the brain. The PET scan measures the activity of the brain. The more active an area of the brain is, the more sugar it uses. In this test, the patient first drinks a glass of sugar water, which contains a chemical tracer which will light up on the scanner. Then, the patient is instructed to complete a memory test or a vocabulary test. After the scan the results are compared to a normal scan.

In Alzheimer's disease, the scan reveals decreases in activity in the areas of the brain that manage memory and in the frontal area which manages thinking and organization. These memory areas of the temporal lobes and frontal lobes are affected first, but as the disease progresses the entire brain reduces function and volume.

A relatively new type of PET scan measures the amount of amyloid in the brain. Patients with Alzheimer's have much more amyloid than normal patients. Recent studies indicate that patients with the mutations for early-onset disease have increased amounts of amyloid ten-to-twenty years before they have symptoms. This confirms the autopsy studies showing that people can have the classic amyloid plaques and tangles without any symptoms of the disease. While it remains uncertain how much burden of amyloid is present before symptoms occur, certainly, the healthier the brain is, via nutrition, education, and a lack of damage from hypertension and injury, the later symptoms can occur.

Current promising research is directed at treatment of these high-risk patients before the amyloid builds up in the brain. Most studies in which the damage has already occurred are much more limited.

Although your first response to this new test may be to troop into the doctor's office and demand an amyloid PET scan, there are several problems with this idea. First, the scan costs about $4,000, and Medicare as well as almost all medical insurance companies, refuse to pay. The reasoning is that the test does not affect treatment. These new scanners are limited in number and are located mostly at medical research centers affiliated with major medical schools. Patient selection is a big factor in determining who is eligible for this test. In 2013, a committee called the Amyloid Imaging Taskforce developed guidelines for physicians to follow regarding appropriate patient selection. [11]

The amyloid PET scan is not indicated for patients with classic clinical criteria for probable Alzheimer's disease (AD). It should not be conducted for persons with no symptoms even though they are worried, or in place of genetic testing for patients at risk of early-onset disease. Further, the test is not recommended for patients who complain of memory impairment but have normal standard-test results.

However, it is recommended for patients with persistent memory cognitive impairment, and patients with progressive dementia who are younger than sixty five. The PET scan is also indicated if a patient's diagnosis is unclear after standard testing. The test should not be administered for non-medical use such as obtaining life insurance or for legal purposes such competency hearings.

Despite these issues, the amyloid PET scan is a breakthrough in many ways. Persons with a high risk of dementia have taken the test at age forty and fifty and shown high amounts of amyloid. These patients can be identified before symptoms develop. They are then eligible for experimental treatments to remove the toxic amyloid. Before-and-after scans can show improvement of amyloid clearance at a fairly accurate level compared to the less accurate the Mini-Mental Status Exam test in which test scores fluctuate. Before the existence of the amyloid PET some patients were misdiagnosed with Alzheimer's disease when they actually had vascular dementia or one of the other dementias. Because their amyloid level was normal, they showed no response to experimental treatments to remove it, which incorrectly made it appear these drugs were ineffective for Alzheimer's, when in fact the patient had been misdiagnosed. To date, the tests for Alzheimer's are expensive, not readily available, and require much cooperation from the patient.

In 2015, the Food and Drug Administration approved Cerebral Assessment Systems Inc's Cognivue device for U.S. distribution. In a non-invasive ten-minute test, this computer-based system measures an individual's cognitive function, and gives primary care doctors a chance to discover cognitive decline at its earliest stage.[12] This test is similar to a video game in which the patient uses a mouse-like device to follow dots and other items seen on a video screen

Cognivue tests do not specifically diagnose Alzheimer's disease or any other dementia. But by yielding a number that quantifies the efficiency of a test subject's cognitive functions, they can detect the beginnings of decline well before more obvious dementia symptoms arise.

Cost of the test has yet to be determined, and it always takes a significant amount of time for Medicare and the insurance companies to decide whether or not they will pay for the exam.

Another new test named Neurotrack has been developed at a private research facility in Palo Alto, California.[13] At the writing of this book, it has not as yet been approved by the FDA. The technology is based on thirty years of research at Emory University. This test does not require language or skills. Patients look at images on a monitor while a camera tracks their eye movements. The test lasts thirty minutes as the patient is shown pictures, one new and the other familiar. Healthy people (and primates, this test was developed using monkeys) look longer at the new image. But Alzheimer's subjects cannot remember familiar images, so they look at new and old images the same amount of time. Ninety two seniors were given the test, and the scores predicted who would develop Alzheimer's within three years. Neurotrack is developing a five-minute version of the test that will be available online once the test can be made available to the general public. For more information, go to www.neurotrack.com.

During a standard workup for dementia, doctors also test for the presence of two infections which can mimic Alzheimer's disease. One is syphilis. Although syphilis is very rare today, it still exists. Third-stage syphilis can affect the brain and cause dementia. Syphilis is caused by bacteria which spread through most tissues of the body, gradually causing damage. That is why most doctors routinely perform a RPR test for syphilis as part of the standard workup for Alzheimer's. Neurosyphilis will show specific changes in reflexes and gait that typical Alzheimer's does not.

I have had more than one angry family member ask me why I thought their mother was a prostitute because I had ordered a test for syphilis. Be assured, it is a part of the standard workup.

The other disease is HIV (AIDS). Patients with long-standing HIV (AIDS) can develop dementia, as the HIV causes a low-grade inflammation of the brain. Patients become confused and disoriented. As the HIV epidemic continues more patients who are older than sixty are being diagnosed, and dementia symptoms attributed to Alzheimer's may actually be due to HIV. The encephalopathy from HIV is usually an end-stage symptom of the disease, and these patients are generally in their last year of life. Patients must sign a form permitting testing for HIV, which needs still more explanation. Patients may refuse, or think they are being accused of infidelity or drug use. Believe me, your doctor is doing his or her job, by being thorough and is not accusing your loved one of anything.

Alzheimer's disease develops over a period of years or decades. Confusion and memory impairment that only lasts a week or two is most likely to be delirium, a brain dysfunction from an infection or a drug reaction. An elderly patient who is usually very clearheaded who presents to the emergency room with confusion may have a urinary tract infection, pneumonia, or a reaction to a prescribed medication. When the infection is treated appropriately, or the offending drug discontinued, the delirium resolves.

HIPAA

Before the patient leaves the doctor's office, be sure to address and sign the appropriate HIPAA paperwork, which allows family members to talk to the physician and nurses with the patient's permission. The Health Insurance Portability and Accountability Act was passed by United States Congress and signed by President Bill Clinton in 1996. This act has many provisions.

Other provisions include measures to safeguard the patient's personal and medical records. The HIPPA act requires a patient sign a written form to authorize family members or care givers to speak to the doctor, nurse or pharmacist about the patient's health. A separate form is needed for each office, pharmacy, and hospital. However, HIPAA has all sorts of unintended consequences. Without a signed form, the staff of a medical office cannot tell family members whether the patient is present or has an appointment. Should the family call the local emergency room to try and locate a missing Alzheimer's patient, they will be advised that patient confidentiality cannot be broken. Legally, the hospital staff cannot say whether or not a patient present.

Although the family can notify the police about a missing person and the police can contact the hospital, most jurisdictions require that someone be missing for more than twenty-four hours before a search begins. This is where an ID bracelet or necklace can become essential for the safety of wandering patients. A few communities have developed a silver alert. This is a quick response system to coordinate an alert with the highway patrol and law enforcement agencies when an impaired elder is reported missing. A silver alert may include radio and television announcements to inform the general public to assist authorities if they have seen the missing elder

Another unintended consequence of HIPAA is the difficulty of bed-bound patients to receive their medications. In the past, family members could pick up the prescription at the pharmacy as well as consult with the pharmacist. Now, every pharmacy must have a signed HIPAA form before they can dispense the medication to anyone other than the patient. This can cause long delays in patients receiving their medication. Some patients can't sign their name because they are paralyzed by a stroke or because they are illiterate or in a coma. Some patients, not just those with dementia, refuse to sign anything.

In most states, physicians are required to report patients with Alzheimer's to the Department of Motor Vehicles. This notification does not automatically rescind the driver's license, but it does mean the DMV will notify the patient to come in and be retested. The testing will include the written exam, the vision exam, and a driving test. In this state, California, the DMV contacts the driver about two to three months after notification.

The rules of the road are encoded in long-term memory, and many of these patients have been driving for more than fifty years. One of my patients who had no short-term memory passed all three sections of the test. That's why it can be very helpful to have the doctor try to persuade the patient that it is unsafe to drive rather than waiting for the DMV retest. I have found that many patients ignore the pleas of their family to stop driving, but will agree with the authority of their doctor.

For more information and help, there are several Alzheimer's chat rooms online, as well as local support groups.

- The Alzheimer's reading room website is www.alz.org. This organization has over four thousand blogs about specific solutions to problems.
- The Alzheimer's Association, founded in 1980, has four thousand local support groups throughout the United States.
- The Area Agency on Aging web site is www.n4A.org.
- The Alzheimer's Disease Education and Referral Center (ADEAR), a branch of the National Institute on Aging can be reached at www.nih.gov/alzheimers. They have multiple fact sheets that can easily be downloaded and printed, all without charge.
- Many local hospitals have Alzheimer's support groups.

- www.alzstore.com has many items to help keep your loved one safe. Many families have to adult-proof their house to prevent dangerous risks. Removing knobs from the stove to prevent fires, changing front door locks with a pass code entry to prevent wandering, and placing childproof locks on the oven and refrigerator doors are just some precautions.

Our family did not know about these resources while Martha Jo was still alive. I wish we had. We would not have felt as isolated, as it is reassuring to know there are millions of other families enduring the same problems. The advice from the Alzheimer' reading room can be very helpful and is available any time of the day or night via the Internet.

CHAPTER THREE

WALKING INTO THE PHARMACY

Currently, four medications have been approved by the Federal Drug Administration for the treatment and management of Alzheimer's disease. Three of them work by the same mechanism and are made by rival pharmaceutical companies. They are:

- Aricept, manufactured by Eisai.
    o Dispensed only in tablet form

- Exelon, manufactured by Novartis.
    o Dispensed as tablet, oral solution, or dermal patch for patients who refuse to take pills or who have trouble swallowing.

- Razadyne, manufactured by Ortho-McNeil
    o Dispensed as either a tablet or oral solution.

All of these drugs are reversible acetyl cholinesterase inhibitors. Just what is a reversible acetyl cholinesterase inhibitor? Computers, iPhones, and all electrical gadgets function with electricity, but contrary to popular belief, our brains and nervous system do not run on electricity.

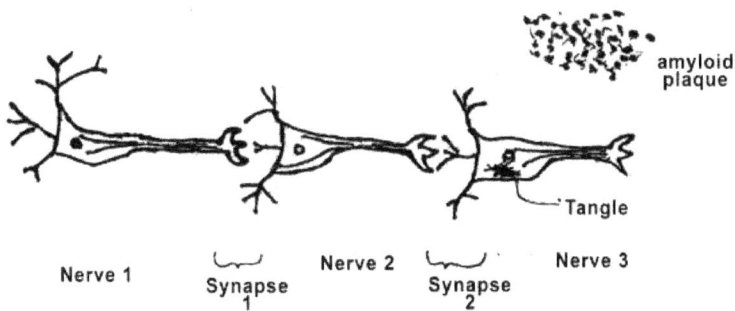

amyloid plaque

Tangle

Nerve 1

Synapse 1

Nerve 2

Synapse 2

Nerve 3

- FIGURE 2 -

Synaptic Space

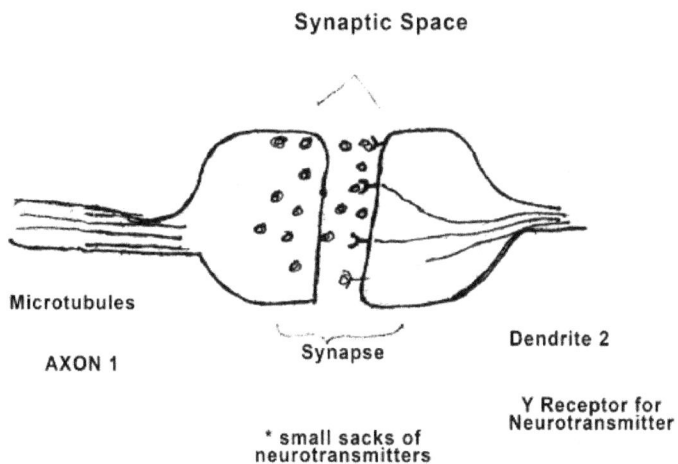

Microtubules

AXON 1

Synapse

Dendrite 2

Y Receptor for Neurotransmitter

* small sacks of neurotransmitters

- FIGURE 3 -
CLOSEUP OF A SYNAPSE

So, how do neurons communicate? As you can see, the neurons don't quite touch each other. A very tiny gap of less than 1/10 of a millimeter lies between the long transmitting axon of nerve #1 and the receiving dendrite of nerve #2, which is covered with microscopic neurotransmitter receptors. When nerve #1 fires, it releases a tiny amount of a chemical called a neurotransmitter. The neurotransmitter floats across the synapse space which is filled with the same mild saline that surrounds all of our cells, and triggers a receptor on the dendrite of nerve #2. Nerve #1 may fire many times, each time releasing the neurotransmitter. After receiving a certain amount of the neurotransmitter, nerve #2 becomes excited and transmits its signal to nerve #3, releasing its own neurotransmitter from its axon to nerve #3.

There are many types of neurotransmitters. In human nerve tissue, the most common is acetylcholine. A decrease of acetylcholine has been discovered in the brains of patients with Alzheimer's disease. Other neurotransmitters in the brain include serotonin, epinephrine, norepinephrine, dopamine, and glutamine. Each chemical is quite distinct from each other. Most neurons use only one type of neurotransmitter. The glutamate system also has a function in memory retention that is similar, but not identical to the cholinergic circuit.

The first studies of how the brain functions at the chemical level used the brains of rats and mice. The amounts of the various neurotransmitters in their brains were measured. This was a very crude estimate, but these studies from the 1970's and 1980's formed the foundation of understanding how the brain works, and how it malfunctions. Slight alterations in the amounts of these neurotransmitters were found to correlate with many serious diseases including Alzheimer's disease.

For instance, low amounts of serotonin are associated with depression. High amounts of dopamine correlate with psychosis, and low amounts of dopamine in certain areas of the brain are found in Parkinson's disease. For years, the medical professional believed depression was just a lack of will power, or schizophrenia was caused by bad parenting. Some people attributed schizophrenia and autism to possession by demons. Now we know there are very real abnormalities in the brain function of afflicted patients, and no amount of will power, prayer, or proper mothering can overcome significant diseases such as autism, schizophrenia, and dementia.

Many different strains of laboratory rats and mice have been deliberately developed over decades with various medical conditions. Some strains of mice are known to develop dementia. As young mice they easily learn new mazes to find food, but when elderly, age two for a mouse, they cannot learn new mazes and forget previously learned ones. Scientists discovered the senile mice had much less of the neurotransmitter acetylcholine than elderly mice which did not show mouse-level traits of dementia.

Using much finer scientific studies, scientists discovered that the brains of Alzheimer's patients also had substantially lower amounts of acetylcholine than normal elderly brains. They reasoned that if the amount of the acetylcholine could be increased in the brain, this might improve symptoms. Although nothing can halt the progressive death of individual neurons, patients may have temporary improvement in memory and cognitive function.

Each time a neuron axon fires, it releases its neurotransmitter. Although it would seem the neurotransmitter would flood the synapse, so it is unable to fire again, similar to a car that can't start with a flooded carburetor, a chemical called an enzyme that is present in the receiving nerve ending breaks down the neurotransmitter. The ending *ase* is used to describe the enzyme that breaks down the neurotransmitter. For example, acetyl cholinesterase is the enzyme that breaks down acetylcholine. If the enzyme is prevented from working, there will be more acetylcholine. This is a double negative; by decreasing the function of the inhibitor enzyme, the amount of the transmitter is increased. All of the drugs for the management of Alzheimer's disease and other mental illness are reversible. The term reversible means the drug blocks the enzyme only for a period of time.

Acetylcholine is also the main neurotransmitter of the nerves located within the walls of the digestive system. It is often referred to as the cholinergic system, whose opposite is the anticholinergic system or adrenergic system, which uses epinephrine as its main neurotransmitter. Too much acetylcholine causes nausea, vomiting, sweating, loss of appetite, diarrhea, and excessive production of mucus in the nose and lungs. Drugs such as Aricept increase acetylcholine in the brain, but also increase acetylcholine in the digestive system. That is why the major side effects of these drugs are nausea, vomiting, diarrhea and excessive production of mucus from the nose and lungs. People take over the counter and prescription anticholinergic drugs to treat these symptoms caused by upper viral illness, viral gastroenteritis, and allergies.

Aricept should not be taken with anticholinergic drugs. The result is like driving a car with one foot on the gas and one on the brake. Anticholinergic drugs are often found in cold and flu treatments, often in combination with antihistamines or other agents. That is why it is important to check with your doctor when using over the counter medications, which can interact with prescriptions.

Many prescription drugs are anticholinergic as well. These include drugs to treat overactive bladder, asthma, COPD, drugs containing Sudafed, and antidepressants in the tricyclic class. So are many of the medicines used to treat diarrhea, irritable bowel syndrome, and dizziness. In addition to the gastrointestinal side effects, they have significant neurological side effects as well. These include sleepiness, confusion, reduced reasoning and reduced short-term memory. These side effects can be confused as being dementia, and these drugs may need to be stopped before proceeding further.

A recent study from 2015 followed three thousand-four hundred men and women age sixty-five and older.[14] They recorded all of the anticholenergic drugs they had taken for ten years before the study started, and the patients' health was followed for an average of seven years. During that time, eight hundred of the patients developed dementia. Persons who used drugs with the strongest anticholinergic effects were more likely to develop dementia than persons who did not use these drugs. Also, people who took the highest doses for the longest time had a 54% higher risk of dementia than patients who took lower doses for short period of time.

How well do these drugs for Alzheimer's disease work? All have been subjected to extensive testing by the manufacturer to be sure there is some benefit.

The pharmaceutical companies are very competitive. If a competitor has a new medication that is generating a lot of revenue, its rivals may create a drug with very similar structure and effectiveness.

However, the results I get from my practice are often quite different from the official studies. About one in ten of my patients will show a marked improvement in memory after taking Aricept for three-to-six months. Sometimes, the patient and family decide to stop the drug after three months because they believe the drug is not working. In several cases, an abrupt decline in function occurred in the week after the drug was stopped. This happens to about half of my patients. Although the patient did not improve while on the medication, they apparently stopped declining as quickly, so the drug did work. Unfortunately, if the drug is restarted again, the level of function does not go back to where it was before the interruption. However, in a situation like this I recommend the drug to be resumed in order to slow the decline of memory.

Martha Jo took Aricept for six months. She had no improvement, and there was no noted change after it was discontinued.

The fourth drug approved to treat Alzheimer's disease is Namenda, manufactured by Forest Laboratories, Inc. Namenda is an N-methyl-D-aspartate receptor antagonist, and is related to dextromethorphan, the DM in Robitussin DM, an over-the-counter cough suppressant, and Amantadine, which is used to treat both influenza and Parkinson's disease.

Namenda can be used alone or in combination with Aricept or any of the other two drugs. However, Namenda's mechanism is very different from these other medications. Namenda does not stop the progressive loss of neurons either. Namenda blocks the nerve receptors from being activated by a small protein, glutamine.

All prescription drugs available in the United States must be approved by the Federal Drug Administration. They are tested extensively, a process that can take more than ten years. Before FDA approval, drugs are tested on thousands of volunteers to be sure they are safe and the symptoms improve. All of these drugs approved for dementia patients have been tested on patients with dementia and healthy volunteers. During the clinical trials, these volunteers have their memory, attention, orientation, and use of language tested before starting the drug. The drug is given to one half of the patients for a period of time, anything between four weeks or even several years. After taking the new medicine for the allotted time the patients are retested. Neither the patient nor the clinician doing the testing knows which patients receive the drug and which are receiving a placebo, or inactive pill. All four FDA approved dementia drugs show test score improvements in patients taking the medication better than chance, and the patients taking the medication show less decline in function.

DEPRESSION

Many other medications are used to treat some of the unpleasant symptoms of Alzheimer's disease. Many patients are depressed years before any mental decline is recognized. My mother would cry for hours for no apparent reason, which was very difficult for our family to witness. Currently, at least twenty antidepressants are on the market and most of them are used to treat depressed patients with dementia. Other symptoms that may improve with the use of antidepressants include, apathy, excessive sleeping up to twenty hours a day, loss of appetite, and temper tantrums.

There are three main groups of antidepressants. The oldest group, first discovered between 1950 and 1980, are the tricyclics. Their chemical structure forms three rings, and they all work in the same way with varying degrees of side effects. As older drugs, they are much cheaper, but also have more side effects and are somewhat less effective than newer medications. However, they can be very useful.

For instance, the tricyclic Elavil has been used successfully for decades. Although it tends to cause sleepiness shortly after taking, this medicine might work very well for a depressed patient who has severe insomnia and can't sleep at night. Elavil would not be a good choice for a depressed patient who sleeps all day and night. Other members of the tricyclic family include Norpramin, Sinequan, Tofranil, Pamelor, Vivactil, and Surmontil.

The tricyclics have similar side effects:

- Dry mouth
- Sedation
- Confusion
- Nausea
- Tremors
- Muscle spasms

Although improved sleep often happens the first night, it takes an average of four-to-six weeks before significant improvement in depression occurs. A major problem with these medications is that if a patient becomes suicidal and overdoses with twenty or more pills, they may succeed in dying. Most doctors do not give any tricyclic antidepressant to dementia patients because all have some degree of anticholinergic effects, reduce memory and can cause confusion. If a patient has been taking these medications for years and develops dementia, the medication should be stopped. Most doctors will not prescribe anti-cholinergic drugs to patients over the age of seventy-five.

In 1984, the first of a new class of antidepressant, Prozac, was released, which revolutionized psychiatry. This new class is named the SSRI class, which is an acronym for selective serotonin reuptake inhibitor. Other members of the class include:

- Celexa
- Lexapro
- Paxil
- Zoloft

These medications create much less sedation side effects and are more activating. Depressed patients seem to develop more energy and, in my opinion, recover faster. The major side effects of this class of medication are nausea, loss of appetite, weight gain, and low sodium in the blood occur. However, these drugs have much fewer problems with low blood pressure than tricyclics, and patients usually do not have the troublesome dry mouth. The SSRI's class of drugs also has a better safety margin. Death from intentional overdoses with these drugs is rare.

That said, the elderly are always at higher risk of dangerous side effects than younger patients. A colleague of mine started an eighty-year-old woman on Paxil, which, at that time, had been on the market for at least ten years. Five days later the patient had a seizure and was taken to the emergency room. The level of salt, or sodium, in her blood was dangerously low and she nearly died. Fortunately, she survived, but this type of traumatic and dangerous side effect is shocking in a drug that is considered safe. All members of the SSRI family can have this rare effect. Just about any medication can have rare but severe complications. Even one aspirin tablet can kill, so can a single penicillin tablet.

Martha Jo took Celexa for years for her depression, and did very well and improved. I told her. "Mom you are doing so much better. You do not get angry any more, you are calm all the time. Last year you would cry for hours at a time and you don't anymore."

"Am I better?" she replied. She seemed unaware how much she had improved.

In 2006, my parents hired an aide to help them at home. My father loves ice cream. My mother asked for some, and it was served to her. Next thing we know, she is eating ice cream every day. But, twenty years prior my mother had been diagnosed with lactose intolerance and she had not consumed milk or ice cream during all that time.

Due to her Alzheimer's, she had forgotten that she had lactose intolerance, and Dad did not remember either. Her doctor attributed her diarrhea to the Celexa and stopped it. The diarrhea continued. She got a colonoscopy. It was completely normal. Finally, after she had suffered for three months with diarrhea, my brother called me. During the course of our conversation, he mentioned that Mom was eating ice cream every day.

"Ice cream." I said. "She isn't supposed to eat that, it gives her severe diarrhea."

Mystery solved. Her diarrhea wasn't caused by Celexa, it was the ice cream. It seems her doctor did not obtain a complete history of allergies. I advise all patients to fill out a small card listing all of their current medications and all of their allergies. Be sure to include what the allergic reaction is. There is a difference between an allergic reaction and a side effect.

An allergic reaction activates the immune system. Rashes, hives, itching, swelling of the tongue and throat, and wheezing are usually allergic reactions.

Sleepiness, insomnia, diarrhea, and nausea are side effects. This means the drug can be given if necessary, and side effects may resolve with a lower dose.

The third class of antidepressants is generally known as the atypicals. They represent a wide variety of chemical forms. Wellbutrin is used frequently for Alzheimer's patients. It also is activating, patients have more energy and are more active during the day. Desyrl causes sleepiness and is sometimes given at bedtime to treat insomnia because it has fewer side effects than other sleep agents. Other antidepressants which are approved for use with Alzheimer's include Effexor, Remeron, and Prestiq.

What patients often don't know is that representatives from various pharmaceutical companies come to doctor's office loaded with large cartons of free samples of the latest medications that they are marketing. They also bring gifts: pens, notepads, brochures, pie, and hats. They may bring lunch for the entire office, and talk to the physicians and physician's assistants about their new medication. Drug representatives need the physician's permission to leave pamphlets in the waiting room about their drug, but the doctor usually doesn't enter their own waiting room and see that literature is there without authorization

The representatives are there to promote sales, and these techniques can be very effective. The plan is to convince the physician to prescribe the new medication and give the patient free samples for the first two weeks or month before they have to pay full price at their neighborhood pharmacy. The new medications are always more expensive than older medications, and often are not on the formularies of the patient's insurance company. Most new drugs take at least a year to get onto insurance formularies.

New launches of drugs also often involve advertisements on television, radio, and in magazines. The success or failure of a new medication is worth millions of dollars to the pharmaceutical company, so it is to their advantage to promote the drug as heavily as possible.

Every doctor I know hates these direct-marketing-to-patient advertisements for prescription drugs. One of my colleagues refuses to prescribe any drug that is promoted by using direct-to-consumer advertising. Until twenty years ago, direct marketing to patients was illegal in all fifty states.

Patients see the ad, and then come to the doctor to request the medication, generally as a question after the primary reason for the appointment has concluded.

My usual reply is, "Why would you want a medicine that costs three times as much as the one you are taking, and that doesn't work as well and has more side effects?"

"Oh, I didn't know," is my patient's usual response.

It can take five or ten minutes to convince the patient they do not need this new drug or that it is not indicated for them. There are several ads for drugs for dementia on the media at this time. It is all right to ask your doctor about the new drug, but please mention this at the start of your visit. Don't just toss out the question at the end of the visit.

ANXIETY

In my opinion, one class of drugs that should not be used for Alzheimer's patients is the Valium family. These include:

- Xanax
- Klonopin
- Halcion
- Ativan
- Librium
- Restoril
- Tranxene

These medications have been used for decades to treat anxiety and insomnia, but all cause memory impairment. There are many stories of healthy individuals who took these medicines before bedtime and awoke the next morning to find a bag of food from a fast food restaurant on their nightstand. They have no memory of leaving the house and going to the store. But the receipt shows the time they were at the store, and there may be crumbs of food on their lips or in the bed.

For someone who already has an impaired memory, these drugs will certainly make them worse. An Alzheimer's patient who is given Valium usually becomes more confused, more disoriented, and more agitated instead of becoming calm. When a patient is diagnosed with dementia or mild cognitive impairment, every effort should be made to take the patient off of the Valium-family drugs to reduce their confusion and memory impairment. Some anti-anxiety medications which are available to replace Valium class members include Buspar, Cymbalta, Effexor, Lexapro, and Zoloft. Neurontin is not classified as an anti-anxiety medication, but it has been used off label for this purpose.

No one should change the dose or discontinue any prescription medication without consulting the prescribing doctor. Abrupt discontinuation of some medications can create life threatening conditions.

My mother was on Klonopin for about ten years. She took her own medications her entire adult life. About 2005, she began to place her daily medications in a large box with small slots for each day's dose. When I came home and actually checked her mediations, I discovered that she was taking much more Klonopin than she was prescribed, and forgetting her blood pressure medications.

Medication errors both deliberate and due to forgetfulness can be deadly. They take a pill, and then ten minutes later they can't remember if they took it and take another. The medication box is supposed to help with this. Open the slot. If the pill you forgot is still there, take it now. If the pill is missing, you already took it. There should be no left over pills in the box at the end of the day.

If your loved one seems confused, double check the prescriptions and make sure they are being taken correctly. Families need to determine when it is no longer safe for a patient to self-medicate. The general answer is when the patient is making major mistakes by taking too much or too little of a prescription, or if they have ever had a deliberate or accidental overdose.

AGITATION

Antipsychotic medicines are often useful for managing agitated, frantic patients. Some patients are extremely restless and continually pace. Many have sun-downing. This is where the patient may be relatively cogent during daytime, but at sunset they become disoriented, confused, agitated, and unable to sleep. They may insist upon wandering through the house, or try to run away into the night screaming or crying.

There are too many antipsychotic medications to list here, but certain ones are used more often and found to be better tolerated than others. Elderly patients are more likely to develop side effects than younger patients, and sometimes the side effects can be worse than the disease. No one drug works for everyone, and often, doctors must use trial-and-error to find a medication that is both tolerated and effective.

Depakote and Lamictal are two antipsychotic medications which seem to be well tolerated and useful for the elderly. Risperdol, Zyprexa, and Seroquel carry black-box warnings of increased risk of death from all causes. Yet, they seem to be the most effective of all in managing the severest symptoms. Despite the risk, these medications may be used for end-stage patients where prolonging life merely prolongs the suffering. Seeing a major improvement in relieving these distressing symptoms, which are not responsive to other treatments, often seems to be worth the risk of sudden death.

An elderly patient of one of my colleagues had been crying non-stop for three days. My colleague had tried three other medications, including Valium, which made her worse. I was on call for my colleague when this episode occurred. The family and the patient were desperate. I ordered 0.25 mg of Risperdol. Thirty minutes later, she stopped crying. The caregivers could not survive seventy-two hours without sleep while their beloved elder seemed to not sleep at all.

Another large class of antipsychotics, of the Thorazine and Haldol family, generally has too many side effects for the elderly. These include sedation, very dry mouth, low blood pressure, and cardiac problems. These medications are also anticholinergic, which are not indicated for long-term use in dementia patients. However, these older medications may prove useful during a short term psychiatric crisis, such as an agitated patient assaulting medical staff in the hospital.

APATHY

Some Alzheimer's patients develop apathy and withdrawal. Many of these patients may sleep twenty hours a day. Ritalin, generally used for hyperactive children can be useful to energize these patients so they can get out of bed. Other members of the methamphetamine family, such as Adderall and Concerta, can also be used for these lethargic patients with good results.

Hundreds of research studies are published every year regarding the possible protective effects of hypertension, diabetes, hyper-cholesterol, and cardiac medications. These clinical trials have followed patients for decades. These trials were designed to determine the incidence of heart attacks, stroke, and deaths from all sources in patients taking long-term, cardiovascular medications. The information in the studies can be reviewed to determine if patients taking the drug had an increased or decreased the risk of dementia. The results are often conflicting. One mega-array tested 1600 medications on cultures of brain cells from mice, and found that 184 may be protective.[15] I think at this time, the results are too mixed to make any recommendation to either prescribe or not prescribe any of the drugs that are used to treat conditions outside their intended use.

HOW MEDICATIONS FOR OTHER AILMENTS PREVENT DEMENTIA

Essentially, any treatment that improves blood flow to the brain such as antihypertensive drugs or diabetic drugs, may improve overall vascular health, and thereby cerebral health, which could improve brain function.

There has been much controversy about the use of the cholesterol lowering drugs called statins to prevent and/or treat Alzheimer's. The literature seems to suggest that statins are ineffective in treating patients who are already diagnosed with Alzheimer's disease.[16] However, statins may be of use to reduce risk or slow down the development of dementia. The mechanism by which statins reduce risk of dementia is twofold.

Excess cholesterol collects inside the walls of arteries. Its presence activates the patient's immune system. The cholesterol deposits are then infiltrated with activated white blood cells which release a variety of chemicals that generally combine to create inflammation. In general, all of this inflammation is toxic to the brain. By reducing inflammation, the damage is reduced. Also, by increasing blood flow through clean arteries, overall brain health is achieved.

About twenty years ago, several clinical studies were completed which showed post-menopausal women had a reduced risk of dementia if they took estrogen replacement for many years. However, subsequent studies denied this protective effect of estrogen.[17] More recent studies showed that the increased risk of breast cancer, stroke, and myocardial infarction from estrogen was of more danger to life and present health than any slight benefit in reducing risk of Alzheimer's, which might not occur for thirty years anyway.

This chapter is limited to currently available FDA approved prescriptions for dementia patients. A physician calculates many factors about prescribing one drug over another. The frequency and severity of side effects are two, how quickly the medicine works is another. Patients who refuse or have difficulty swallowing pills may do better with a patch which is applied to the skin. Drugs applied to the skin usually have fewer side effects. Many tell me capsules slide down easier than pills. A few of these medicines are available as a liquid. Cost is a major factor for many families.

Don't be afraid to talk to your doctor. He or she might think that the medicine isn't working, when it is in fact not being given at all. Doctors are aware of this difficulty, so please don't feel embarrassed. Physicians often try to obtain free samples supplied by pharmaceutical representatives. Samples can be very useful in the short-term with regard to possible side effects and patient tolerance. However, the physician can only dispense a few weeks of worth of samples, and then the patient must assume the cost. Most doctors use just one or two members of a class of drugs because they have used them frequently and had good results.

Lastly, the new drugs promoted by commercials may have never been used by the physician. Most doctors I know don't watch much television and may not know about drugs mentioned on TV. Once a patient asked me about a medicine recommended by Dr. Oz.

"Who is he, is that the same as the Wizard of Oz?" I replied. About a month later I had the afternoon off, and intentionally watched his show so I would know what my patients were talking about.

Computers have made prescribing safer. A troublesome problem is a patient who is seeing several different doctors. These doctors may be unaware of each other, and prescribe conflicting drugs, or are prescribing the same drug in different doses. Today, the pharmacy software can often pick this up and alert the physician. I had at least one patient who was taking Valium, Xanax and Halcion prescribed by three different doctors. She was not aware the three medicines were in the same family and she was at high risk for a near fatal overdose or car accident. Of course drugs in the valium family and pain medicines can be abused, sold, or taken in order to get a high, which is why some states have placed more restrictions on them. This is another reason it is so important to keep a current list of all medicines from all doctors and show it to each one at every visit.

A useful guide for doctors, nurses, and all medical caregivers who treat the elderly is the Beers Criteria for Potentially Inappropriate Medication Use in Older Adults. It was created by the American Geriatrics Society. It was recently updated in 2012. This sixteen page guide has recommendations for or against several hundred prescriptions for the elderly and it can be downloaded from the internet at www.healthimaging.org.

CHAPTER FOUR

WALKING INTO THE COURTHOUSE

As I am a physician, I cannot offer legal advice. However, at the time you or your loved one is diagnosed with Alzheimer's disease, several legal issues should be addressed to determine whether or not they are applicable in your state or country. Please consult an attorney who is licensed in your state, is familiar with estate planning and elder care, and who can answer your questions and provide guidance.

Here are some general guidelines and a few issues to think about.

PERSONAL FINANCES

One of the most important things to do while the patient is still competent is to write a will or update it. Another task is to add a trusted family member to bank accounts and as a signer on a credit card. The family member can then pay the bills with the patient's own money.

If the patient is sole owner of a car or house, the spouse, adult child, or other family member could be added as co-owner.

If the patient has been contemplating a family trust, this is the time to set one up. If not, then this is the time to bring up the subject. Generally, a family trust is a method of moving assets to the next generation with a minimum of estate taxes. If the patient owns a business, a farm, or has a significant amount of assets, a family trust might be useful. However, even people without Alzheimer's may balk at the idea of a family trust. They may feel afraid of losing control of their life and finances. A major fear is that their relatives may sell their house and belongings and put them in a care facility against their will.

Another solution would be to appoint a non-interested third party, such as a trust officer from their bank or financial advisors to serve as conservator, who can take control of the patient's finances after the patient is declared incompetent by one or two different physicians. The trust officer then has access to the patient's finances and can pay bills. These trust officers must qualify by taking many accredited accounting courses and be bonded.

STATE AND FEDERAL DISABILITY

If the patient is working at the time of diagnosis, he or she may qualify for state disability. The employer may have a disability insurance policy.

The Consolidated Omnibus Budget Reconciliation Act (COBRA) gives workers and their families who lose their health benefits the right to choose to continue group health benefits provided by their group health plan for limited periods of time under certain circumstances such as voluntary or involuntary job loss, reduction in the hours worked, transition between jobs, death, divorce, and other life events. More information on COBRA benefits can be found on the Department of Labor website, www.dol.gov. This can be a life saver for patients with disease who were still working at the time of diagnosis. Another source of possible income is Social Security Disability Income (SSDI). A person needs to have a certain number of work credits to qualify. Visit your local Social Security office for general information and to apply. They now have a web page available and many questions and forms can be obtained on line.

If the patient does not have enough work credits to qualify for SSDI, he or she may qualify for Supplemental Security Income (SSI) which is based on financial need. They can qualify for SSI disability after they have been disabled for two years. SSI disability does not require a person to be sixty-five years of age, but they must be a legal resident of the US.

HEALTH INSURANCE & MEDICARE

The ACA (Affordable Care Act), passed in 2012, has changed the ability of patients to obtain health care. Before the ACA a person could not obtain health insurance at any price if they had certain pre-existing health conditions. Now a person who is younger than sixty-five with a diagnosis of dementia can get insurance. Previously, medical insurance companies refused to insure patients with a history of cancer, stroke, dementia of any kind, diabetes, most heart conditions, and a huge list of other health ailments.

Many people are surprised to hear that Medicare does not pay for long-term nursing home care or assisted living. Currently Medicare will pay for one hundred days of skilled nursing care if the patient was admitted to a hospital for three days prior to the nursing home, but there are many restrictions about coverage. You can check your local Medicare website, or discuss with a social worker or patient care coordinator.

Patients can buy insurance for long-term assisted living and skilled nursing. These policies tend to be very expensive, and multiple medical conditions will cause the application to be denied. Each insurance company makes its own rules; the reasons for refusal of long-term care insurance include a positive test for HIV, a history of cancer, a history of drug or alcohol abuse, the diagnosis of a degenerative neurological diseases such as Parkinson's disease, stroke, multiple sclerosis, dementia of any cause, and ALS, having a prior admission to a nursing home or assisted living, or needing assistance with activities of daily living (ADL) such as bathing, dressing, movement, or eating. If a person has any of these situations it is too late to sign up for supplemental long-term care policies.

Medicare will pay for skilled nursing care if the patient was admitted to an acute care facility, a hospital, and stayed there for at least seventy-two hours. The diagnosis must be one that requires acute hospitalization, and the treating physician must request the transfer. The nursing home must have room, and has final say about accepting the patient. Medicare generally does not pay the entire rate, basing their payments in a sliding scale fashion. There are a variety of charges besides the room rate. Patients are charged for every item used such as drugs, bandages, nursing care, and therapy.

All patients admitted to an acute care hospital are given an acuity of care evaluation. This means that the patient must have a medical condition which meets the criteria of hospital admission. For example, pneumonia of one lung by itself is not criteria for admission. The majority of patients with pneumonia can be managed at home on oral antibiotics. The presence of a fever or an elevated white count usually is not criteria by themselves. The criteria for admission for pneumonia include a low oxygen level in the blood, severe shortness of breath, accompanying dehydration, low blood pressure, severe nausea and vomiting that prevent the person from taking fluids and medication, and failure of the pneumonia to resolve with oral antibiotics.

Every admission requires a list of qualifying conditions, and doctors are very familiar with all of them. Each hospital has a Medicare compliance officer, usually an RN who interacts with the physicians to ensure the correct Medicare payment codes are listed to increase the likelihood that Medicare will pay the bill.

Medicare audits each admission. If the Medicare auditor believes that the patient doesn't meet criteria, Medicare refuses to pay the bill. Then the hospital charges the patient. But, the patient, or POA (power of attorney), must sign a form, one of the dozens, to be filled out upon admission, stating that they accept financial responsibility for payment if Medicare or other insurance refuse coverage. Many patients have been unpleasantly surprised by bills as high as $500,000.

Don't panic. Talk to the doctor. Perhaps some other Medicare codes could be used which apply to the situation. Medicare rules can seem arbitrary and bizarre. A primary diagnosis of dehydration and secondary diagnosis of pneumonia can pay twice as much as a primary diagnosis of pneumonia and secondary dehydration. The average patient bill varies greatly from one region to another, but is generally much higher in cities than in rural areas.

Although families are often in distress when a loved one continually wanders or puts him or herself at risk, unfortunately, they cannot have the patient admitted to the hospital without this specific acuity of care criteria.

The family of one of my patients demanded that I admit the patient to the hospital for three days so that Medicare would pick up the first one hundred days of skilled nursing care. When I had to tell them that I could not because their loved one did not meet the criteria for admission, they threatened to sue me, and then fired me. They brought another doctor in to admit the patient, who also denied admission.

Families are often in crisis. One of my patients with early disease placed dirty dishes into the oven (believing the oven to be a dish washer) and turned on the oven, causing a fire. The patient and hysterical family went to the local emergency room at midnight and demanded the patient be admitted to the hospital. Again, because the patient did not meet Medicare's medical criteria for admission, they were refused. That unhappy family returned home and started looking for assisted living the next morning.

I have admitted dementia patients to the hospital for acute medical conditions and found no family answers the phone number listed, and no family members can be located. The patient is confused, sometimes homeless or wandering. The patient stayed at the hospital for many days or even weeks until the family members returned from wherever they were.

Medicare does not pay for everything. In general it pays eighty percent of expenses such as medications, physician payments, and treatments. Medicare patients can buy supplemental insurance to fill in this so called Medi-gap. There are many advertisements on television, offers in the mail, and phone calls selling these policies. Applications may be limited to an open enrollment period, generally at the time of their sixty-fifth birthday, and the first of the New Year. These policies do cost money, but in general they save more than they cost. The cost varies with the amount of covered benefits, and varies from one county to another and one company from another.

MEDICAID

All fifty states have Medicaid, which is designed to assist low income patients, currently defined as having an income of less than 138% of the poverty level. This value is calculated each year. Unlike Medicare, Medicaid does pay for nursing home care. Most dementia patients older than sixty-five may qualify for both Medicare and Medicaid, which together would pay almost all expenses. However Medicaid, which is a federal and state funded entitlement program established in 1963, was specifically designed for low income patients. Initially, patients had to divest their assets such as a house, car, or business in order to qualify for Medicaid, as assets could not be above a certain amount to qualify for the program.

For decades, the most common cause of personal bankruptcy has been severe illness. After becoming injured or ill, the person is not able to work. Without any income, they can't pay the health insurance premiums or pay for medical care either. Since about 1993 people no longer face having to sell their house, car, and other assets to qualify for Medicaid. Instead, Medicaid is required to seek repayment for some of the expenses through the Estate Recovery Program.[18] This means the federal government and state can place a lien on the estate of the patient after the patient's death. Generally, this lien was for costs associated with skilled nursing facilities.

An exception is that if the Medicaid recipient has a child less than twenty-one years of age, or a disabled family member living at their house then the state cannot file the lien for repayment until the minor is older than twenty-one, or when the disabled member dies or moves out.

Today, the Affordable Care Act has changed this. Some Medicaid patients are enrolled in HMO's (Health Management Organizations). The state and federal government pay a premium to the HMO each month, whether the patient is seen or not. Under traditional Medicaid, the various vendors were paid at a fee for service. So, if a patient had no medical visits or costs, there was nothing to bill. In ten states, including California, the state may place a lien of the estate of the patient for the return of all premiums paid to the HMO after age fifty-five for the purpose of repayment of nursing home costs. These premiums may be $600 each month, which adds up to $7000 each year.

Patients can apply for Medicaid and ACA at an ACA center or on-line. Sometimes the process is straight forward, and sometimes it can be difficult. The main caretaker often needs to contact an attorney to represent them in qualifying for SSI disability, Medicaid, or Medicare if the person is younger than sixty-five. These proceedings may take many months or years, and are hard on the nerves. Essentially every major city in the United States has ads on television from plaintiff attorneys, and they often have large ads in the phone book telling if they do disability work or Medicaid. The social worker at the hospital may have some suggestions.

POWER OF ATTORNEY

The next step is obtaining a power of attorney. This form must be completed when the dementia patient is still competent to manage their affairs. If the treating physician believes the person is not competent to understand and sign the Power of Attorney, the family must petition the county court for guardianship and conservatorship.

This can be a very burdensome process which could take several months to accomplish. It is much easier to sign Power of Attorney, especially for spouses early, than go to court later.

In fact, for most patients over the age of sixty, I advise completing the Power of Attorney now. You never know when or if you will become incapacitated.

A close family member had a massive stroke in his late fifties. He had never discussed his wishes about code status, must less had named a POA. A power of attorney permits a person to name a relative to manage their financial affairs if they become incompetent or unable to manage their own affairs. Married persons generally name their spouse if the spouse is able to do so. If there is no competent spouse, an adult child or an adult grandchild may be named. Other possible relatives include nieces, nephews, and cousins.

The person named as power of attorney must be well enough to manage the patient's affairs and also must agree to do it. They are not required to live in the same state. An attorney can draw up the document. The patient and the chosen power of attorney must sign the document and have it notarized.

Although it is possible to download a power of attorney form on line, please be aware that it can be contested, especially if the person named as power of attorney is not related to the patient, or seems to be exploiting the patient.

There are two types of powers of attorney(POA), medical and financial. The medical POA allows the POA to speak to the doctor, make medical decisions, and sign consent for medical procedures. It also allows them to obtain medical records.

The financial POA allows the person named POA to access bank accounts, authorizes them to sell assets to pay bills if needed, file and sign state and federal taxes, and sue creditors to reach a settled amount. Further, the financial POA can file for social security, social security disability, and health insurance on behalf of the patient. He or she can also arrange for, and sign contracts such as those for an in-home caretaker.

In most states, it is illegal for physicians to also be the POA for a patient, as it is considered to be a breach of medical ethics. The POA must be someone who has shown themselves to be trustworthy, as they will have access to all financial and personal business. Extreme care should be taken when considering who should have power of attorney because, sadly, every town has its stories of the dishonest POA.

GUARDIANSHIP AND CONSERVATORSHIP

In the absence of a valid POA, then a family member must request guardianship and conservatorship. If no relative can be found or will volunteer, then the county court will appoint a guardian. Generally, this would be a court-appointed attorney who may have several other wards in the county. A court-appointed guardian does not work for free. He or she must visit the ward at least once a year and usually charges by the hour for his work on behalf of the ward. This could be up to three hundred or more dollars an hour, plus expenses such as travel to visit the ward. Payment comes from the ward, unless they are indigent, in which the state pays out of a fund.

Guardian means being legally responsible for someone. Conservancy means being able to handle their financial affairs. The applicant will need a different attorney to represent them as a conservator. Again, the county court will appoint an attorney to represent the patient. Now, there are two attorneys, each charging the patient for their fees and expenses.

There are extensive documents to be completed, as well as an inventory of the patient's assets. There will be a court hearing. A physician must conduct an examination to determine if they are competent.

While this book is about dementia, many patients suffer from long-standing mental illness, brain trauma, or mental retardation and require guardianship. For patients with dementia, their primary care physician can sign the physician's document. If incompetency is due to mental illness, the medical document needs to be completed by a psychiatrist or a neuropsychologist. Usually, medical insurance will not pay for a competency evaluation for legal purposes because they only pay for actually treatment of disease. The cost of filing for guardianship and conservatorship varies, but expect at least ten thousand dollars or more to be paid by the patient or family.

The state requires the conservator to locate and list the patient's assets and fill out the various accounting forms. This inventory is usually due within ninety days. All of the patient's assets must be accounted for with receipts. A budget must be presented to the court for the next year. After one year, the entire records of all expenses, debt, and debt payments must be filed by a certain deadline. It is a lot of work.

Usually, a minimum of thirty days elapses between filing for guardianship and receiving temporary guardianship. In the meantime, the collection agencies keep calling, although due to confidentiality, they can only speak to the patient. The unopened mail piles up, as it is illegal to open another person's mail.

If you are a direct relative or friend of a patient who is waiting for conservatorship, never pay a bill for the patient out of your own account. Then the collection agencies can sue you because the paid bill shows that you have accepted financial responsibility for the patient.

ELDER ABUSE

An unpleasant way to walk into the courthouse is to be under arrest, and accused of elder abuse or even manslaughter.

A very sad case here in California concerned an elderly woman who had become bedbound and developed large bed sores. She absolutely insisted she was not to be taken to the hospital or see a doctor. She had one full-time caretaker, her niece, who did as she was told. Eventually, the bedsores became severely infected. The patient became unconscious from the infection and was finally taken to the local emergency room where she died.

The unpaid niece, who spent three years caring for her aunt was arrested and charged with elder abuse, neglect, and manslaughter. The niece was in county prison for a year, until found not guilty at her trial. Had she been convicted, she would have faced seven years to life in prison.

Elder abuse law varies from one state to another. The state bar association is a good source of information about your state's laws.

The following information is from the state of California website, "What should I know about Elder Abuse?" at www.ca.gov

Elder abuse is defined as neglect, exploitation, painful, or harmful mistreatment of anyone age sixty-five or older or anyone aged eighteen to sixty-four who is a dependent adult. This includes physical violence, psychological abuse, isolation, abandonment, and abduction. This also includes crimes, such as criminal fraud, theft, and identity theft. No one can strike the elder, withhold food, place the patient in a locked room, or tie them into a bed which is considered to be false imprisonment. It is illegal to deny medical care or fail to give the patient their prescription medications. It is illegal to fail to attend to bedsores or injury. Physicians and nurses are mandatory reporters of suspected abuse. They must report suspected abuse, generally to

Adult Protective Services. Failure to report can be a crime for mandatory reports. Caregivers, paid or unpaid are required to report if they have accepted responsibility for a person. This includes reporting situations occurring in Assisted Living or Skilled Nursing situations. If the patient is a resident of a long term care facility, there may be a local ombudsman. If the situation involves danger, call 911. When the police arrive, explain what happened. It is possible to obtain an Emergency Protective order which legally prohibits the suspected abuser from coming near the patient and or caregiver, similar to a temporary restraining order. Other agencies to contact include the local city police, the county police and the state attorney general In California, http://ag.ca.gov/bmfea/pdfs/citizens_guide.pdf provides general information and guidelines on what to do if you suspect or are a victim of elder abuse.

The National Center on Elder Abuse http://www.ncea.aoa.gov/ provides more information and resources. Your state also may have a bureau of Medicaid fraud and elder abuse hotline.

In addition to physical and psychological mistreatment, financial exploitation of elders is also considered to be elder abuse. Cases of elder abuse are exploding in this country, and are not restricted to patients diagnosed with dementia. Elders at high risk of exploitation are persons who are recently bereaved, abusers of alcohol or drugs, socially isolated, and suffering from depression or mental illness. Of all elder abuse cases reported, thirty percent were for financial exploitation.

The Elder Investment Fraud and Financial Exploitation Prevention Program (EIFFE) in partnership with the American Bar Association, educates elders and well as attorneys and financial investors.

Some common schemes include caregivers or family members using their elder's assets for their own gain, such as retirement funds and social security checks, as well as writing checks to themselves when they know the elder has poor eyesight and memory. Trusted financial advisors may sell inappropriate annuities or mutual funds used to generate huge fees. Then there are scams by phone, email, or mail. Officers and employees of financial institutions also must report known or suspected financial elder abuse.

My parents planned ahead. They had a family trust completed by 1998. They both completed living wills and named each other power of attorney decades before the need arose. I am very thankful to them for their efforts, as my brother and I never needed to decide for them about their care and finances. Most families are not so fortunate.

Contemplating your own death and making end of life decisions is an unpleasant topic. Worse is never discussing it at all, leaving family members confused and undecided. I have been at the bedside of many patients in the intensive care unit advising a family about their dying relative's care. The family is often bitterly divided. Most physicians ask the family to appoint one spokesperson to represent the family. The doctor simply does not have the time to relate to each family member the same information about their relative. In cases where no family can be located, or the family cannot make a unified decision, each hospital has a Medical Ethics committee which can provide counseling about the situation, and make a final decision about medical care for incompetent, or unconscious patients.

Walking into a Court House or attorney's office is intimidating, frightening, and expensive. Not walking into the Court house or attorney's office can result in charges of elder abuse, arrest, bankruptcy, unnecessary and painful medical procedures, and suffering of both patients and their families.

CHAPTER FIVE

WALKING INTO THE HEALTH FOOD STORE

Martha Jo never walked into a health food store in her life. Maybe she should have. I know I never walked into one until five years ago. I was put off by the lack of scientific data about most claims about various diets and health, and both of us ate the standard American diet. In an effort to lose weight twenty years ago, I stopped eating sugary foods, and stopped eating saturated fat from meats and eggs because of its link to coronary artery disease. In recent years, significant new results between diet and prevention of dementia have been found.

In a July 2013 report, the Physicians Committee for Responsible Medicine, discussed a correlation of diet and exercise to the development of dementia.[19] This report was presented at the International Conference on Nutrition and the Brain. Persons who follow these recommendations are expected to reduce their risk of developing Alzheimer's by as much as fifty percent. The committee's recommendations included:

MINIMIZE FOODS HIGH IN SATURATED AND TRANS FATS AND MINERALS.

Unsaturated fat is liquid at room temperature. Common sources include olive oil, canola, vegetable, and corn oil. Saturated fat is solid at room temperatures. It is found in full fat dairy products, butter, lard, red meat, and meats ground together with fat such as sausage and hamburgers.

However two plant sources of saturated fat include palm oil and coconut oil. Trans fats occur naturally in tiny amounts in dairy and meat. Trans fats are added as preservatives for food containing fat, so that foods do not go rancid for a much longer period of time. Most food labels describe trans fats as partially hydrogenated oils. During the production of trans fats, hydrogen atoms are added to unsaturated fats. They preserve freshness in pastries and the icing on the pastries, especially the type found in wrappers and boxes. Trans fats are added to many snacks to give them a long shelf life. This includes potato, cheese, and corn chips. Trans fats are used to preserve the oil in microwave popcorn. They prolong the life of deep fat fryers, so French fries, doughnuts, and fried chicken and fish can absorb trans fats during frying.

Trans fats also seem to be the worst offender of the three types of fat in the development of atherosclerosis and dementia. Trans fats lower HDL, the good cholesterol, and increase LDL the bad cholesterol. Because of bad publicity, several retail outlets and restaurants have publically committed to stopping the use of trans fats in their foods. In 2015, the FDA recommended phasing out the use of trans fats within three years. However, stopping the use of all trans fats could result in an increase of food poisoning, and the marked increase of spoiled foods.

Researchers followed adult volunteers for four years. Those who ate the most saturated fat each day were two to three times more likely to develop Alzheimer's disease compared to those who ate much less. Patients with total blood cholesterol levels above 250 mg/dl had a fifty percent higher risk of developing Alzheimer's disease compared to patients whose blood level was less than 200 mg/dl.

The committee and others have noted that minerals such as iron and copper are very strong oxidizers meaning that they combine readily with oxygen. Excess amounts of both minerals can be stored in the brain as well as bone marrow and liver. It is possible that excessive amounts of these minerals may damage the brain due to oxidative stress.

Some vitamin tablets contain copper and iron. Other sources include liver and red meat. Dates from palm trees are also a rare plant-based source of iron. Cooking food in a cast iron skillet can increase iron content in foods. High copper amounts are present in oysters, kale, and mushrooms. It is true both copper and iron are required as trace elements, but an excess of these minerals can cause damage. Only persons who have low iron levels as determined by their doctor should take iron supplements.

A major public scare occurred thirty years ago when research determined that Alzheimer's patients had higher levels of aluminum in their brains than controls. Many families threw away their aluminum cookware for fear that food cooked in aluminum pots and pans could absorb the aluminum. Additional studies concluded that aluminum is not absorbed in cooking.

However, the committee has recommended the avoidance of anti-acids, baking powder, and vitamins that contain aluminum. Of note, most commercial pastries contain aluminum from the baking powder. Some patients have gone so far to not use antiperspirants which contain aluminum chloride, but there have been no definite studies that aluminum chloride is absorbed through the skin.

EAT A DIET HIGH IN FRUITS, NUTS, VEGETABLES, VITAMINS B-12 AND D

The committee recommends a diet high in vegetables, beans, fruits and whole grains such as whole wheat and brown rice.

The committee also recommends the consumption of fifteen milligrams of vitamin E a day. One ounce of nuts or seeds each day contains about 5 mg. Vitamin E is also present in tomatoes, spinach, avocadoes, and mangos. Many clinicians note that taking a vitamin pill is a very different thing from eating fresh fruits and vegetables. These whole natural foods may contain other nutrients that have not been discovered yet. When studies have been conducted about the effect of vitamins they are consumed as a tablet and not in their natural state.

A separate study from from Maurice Dysken MD followed six

hundred thirteen patients who were already diagnosed with dementia, who were given supplements of vitamin E.[20] During follow up of an average of two years, researchers found that the treated patients did have a slowing of the decline associated with dementia compared to those who did not take the supplement.

The committee recommended a daily intake of 2.4 mcg of vitamin B-12. It is vital in the production of red blood cells, replication of all cells, and maintaining the health of neurons. Symptoms of low vitamin B-12 levels include anemia, numbness and tingling of the hands and feet due to damage to nerve cells, weakness of muscles, confusion, and damage to the nerve cells located in the retina of the eye. Vitamin B-12 is present only from animal sources, especially high in fish, fish oil, liver and kidney. Vegans and vegetarians are strongly advised to take supplemental B-12. Some people lack the intrinsic factor which is necessary to absorb vitamin B-12, which results in these symptoms despite an adequate intake. Patients with this condition, called pernicious anemia, require injections of B-12 for life.

The last committee recommendation is to complete forty minutes of brisk walking or other aerobic exercise three times per week.

Martha Jo did not follow any of the committee's recommendations. She ate sausages and saturated fat. She did not eat fish or take vitamins. Other than the tomatoes she grew in her garden, she ate canned vegetables which are lower in nutrition than fresh, and did not like salad. The only exercise she got was playing golf once a week and she had stopped even that about ten years before her diagnosis.

In a study from 2014, researchers tested the blood levels of vitamin D in 1,658 adults who did not have dementia.[21] The patients were followed for an average of five-and-a-half years. During that time, 102 members of the group developed Alzheimer's disease. Results revealed that the participants with the lowest amounts of vitamin D were much more likely to develop dementia than those who had sufficient concentrations in their blood. Natural sources of Vitamin D are mostly animal based, egg yolks, fish, fish oil, liver, cheese. There is significant amount of vitamin D in mushrooms. People can make their own vitamin D from exposure of skin to sunlight. During the winter, and individuals with dark skin can have very low vitamin D levels.

I live in central California which has plenty of sunshine, and I was shocked when several of my patients had non-detectable levels of Vitamin D. It seems that many people, especially the elderly are not exposed to sunshine at all. Very low Vitamin D levels are rampant in persons who live in assisted living and nursing homes. Beside the role of Vitamin D in the healthy function of nerves, it is essential in the health of bones and treatment and prevention of osteoporosis. Recently, very low levels of Vitamin D have been associated with fibromyalgia.

GINKGO BILOBA

Other scientific studies have been conducted on Ginkgo biloba. For thousands of years, the leaves of the ginkgo tree have been used as a tea and an herbal remedy in Chinese medicine to improve mental function. These studies tried to determine whether or not Ginkgo was of any value in either preventing or delaying dementia as well as a treatment for patients who had been diagnosed.

A study published in Phytomedicine gave patients already diagnosed with Alzheimer's disease Ginkgo biloba in addition to the standard cholinesterase inhibitors.[22] Ginkgo was given for a period of one year to 29 patients, and the remaining 799 in the group received only the cholinesterase inhibitors. Follow-up testing did not show any statistically significant change. A different study found no benefit to healthy adults taking Ginkgo biloba to prevent dementia. [23]

FISH AND OMEGA-THREE FISH OIL

More than twenty large-scale studies have been conducted to investigate the relation between dementia and the consumption of fish and omega-three fish oil. A mega-analysis conducted by Cederholm in Sweden combined results from dozens of studies to make their conclusions.[24] The longest studies followed healthy elders who ate fish at least once a week for time frames that ranged from two to seven years. Although most of these studies indicated a reduced risk of Alzheimer's with weekly fish consumption, at least three additional studies showed there was no relation between eating fish and cognition. The studies involving treating persons already diagnosed with Alzheimer's disease with omega-three oil have been disappointing. Dozens of studies about the effectiveness of omega-three fish oil given to healthy elders shows conflicting evidence about reducing the risk of dementia.

Many persons have reduced fish consumption in the past several years due to reports of mercury contamination. Following a massive earthquake and tsunami in Fukushima Japan, millions of gallons of radioactive contaminated water was returned to the Pacific Ocean. It is possible the radioactive particles have entered the food chain of the Northern Pacific, and into far-ranging fish such as salmon and tuna.

CARNITINE

Acetyl-L-carnitine has a reputation as being marketed as the cure-all for human diseases, and there are many claims regarding its benefit for overall brain health and treatment of dementia.

Carnitine is a natural substance made in the body, and it does increase acetylcholine release and has several other enzymatic functions. Supplements of carnitine have been available in health food stores for decades. It has been studied for both treatment and prevention of brain health and cardiovascular disease. Studies conducted on rats indicate that long-term use of carnitine improved their memory.

An online search will find hundreds of references and many sales pitches. An older study in Neurology treated sixty-three patients diagnosed with Alzheimer's disease with two grams of L-carnitine for one year and compared their tests results with sixty-seven Alzheimer's patients treated with placebo.[25] Fourteen tests of memory, depression and learning were completed before the start of the study and after one year. Both patients taking carnitine and placebo performed worse after one year, however, the decline in test scores was much less in the patients treated with carnitine. Statistical analysis shows this to be a significant difference.

SUPERFOODS

I first heard the term superfood about five years ago. My nutrition class in medical school thirty years ago certainly never mentioned them. A review of the internet shows dozens of foods being called superfoods and marketed as such. The term seems to be a food that has very high levels of vitamins, antioxidants, and minerals for health. Lists vary, but kale and blueberries appear on most. Now kale salads are appearing everywhere and kale chips also. Another unlikely superfood is dark chocolate, which I find to be amazing. Chocolate has always been the first food banned in all diets, and attributed to be the culprit behind teen age acne, diabetes, and high cholesterol. Now it is a health food! It has a strong anti-oxidant effect. It contains resveratrol and flavanoids which lower LDL, the bad form of cholesterol. It contains mono-unsaturated fats similar to coconut oil. Dark chocolate does not contain milk and most types are seventy percent cacao.

One superfood mentioned in the scientific literature is curry, which is derived from tumeric in the ginger family. Several decades ago some demographers noted a slightly lower incidence of dementia in the citizens of India. The association seemed to be based on curry consumption, which is very high in this culture. Tumeric by itself is a strong anti-inflammatory. Dr. James Duke, PhD has produced extensive information about nutrition. He found fifty studies about the use of tumeric and Alzheimer's disease.[26] It was found to block the formation of beta-amyloid 42 and has also been used to treat arthritis for centuries. My mother never ate Chinese or Indian food in her entire life.

Another candidate as a superfood is coconut oil. It is one of two (the other is palm oil) of a saturated fat from a plant source. It has no cholesterol and contains medium chain triglycerides. It is solid at room temperature. There is now a kiosk at my health food store selling coconut oil. It comes in capsules and also in various amounts. One can stir a teaspoon of it into a cup of hot coffee, add to hot oatmeal or spread it on toast. It can be mixed with peanut butter, protein powders, cocoa and used in cooking replacing butter.

A pediatrician named Mary Newport, M.D. wrote a book titled

Alzheimer's Disease: What if there was a cure?[27] She gave her husband a daily dose of coconut oil after his diagnosis of Alzheimer's. He showed improvement after the first dose, and his improvement was sustained. Dr. Newport's book has only one patient, her husband, but there are some clinical trials that are being started to see if other Alzheimer's patients benefit as well as Mary's husband. It has been noted that because coconut oil cannot be patented by the pharmaceutical companies, research funding is limited. However, coconut oil is non-toxic and I know many people are using it based on her book.

ARE GRAINS TOXIC?

Every day on television, there are countless talk shows, cooking programs and medical interview segments that discuss the link between the poor diet of Americans and their resulting poor health. The average American eats too much salt, too much sugar, processed foods and junk food that contain no nutrition and empty calories. The result is rampant obesity, diabetes mellitus, auto immune disease, and coronary artery disease. One physician, Dr. David Perlmutter, a neurologist, has written a book titled *Grain Brain: The Surprising Truth about Wheat, Carbs, and Sugar—your Brain's Silent Killers.*[28] I recommend his book for readers interested in learning more about the effect of grains on brain health.

Some individuals have created the so-called Paleolithic diet. This is believed to be the diet of our ancestors. Our ancestors lived as hunters and gatherers; a lifestyle a few cultures continue. However, they also lived in a large variety of climates, from the tropics to the artic, clearly consuming a myriad of foods. There is much disagreement about this diet, such as are white potatoes and sweet potatoes allowed, and what about lentils. This diet is very difficult to follow, and we really do not know for sure what our ancestors ate.

GLUTEN

My patients often ask me my opinion about a gluten free diet. Gluten is one protein found in wheat, barley, and rye, but not in rice or corn. Gluten is present in both whole wheat flour and white flour. It is also an additive and appears in several foods one would not expect such as mustard. After reading extensively, I do have some recommendations. If the patient has been diagnosed with Irritable Bowel Syndrome with bloating, gas, and diarrhea I strongly recommend giving a gluten free diet a trial run of at least three months. Likewise, I recommend it for patients with auto-immune disease such as thyroiditis or rheumatoid arthritis, migraine headaches, or poorly controlled diabetes. I also recommend it to patients diagnosed with mild cognitive impairment. If a patient with Alzheimer's is agreeable I would try it out as well. It cannot possibly hurt a person and may be of benefit. It will be many years until the results of more clinical trials can be completed. I do not recommend a gluten free diet for everyone. This is very unrealistic. A gluten free diet is expensive. Not very many people can afford lots of fresh vegetables and lean meats. The Italians are not going to stop eating pasta and the French are not going to give up croissants and bread. Fully 25% of humanity faces food insecurity and are certainly not going to decline a twenty-pound bag of white flour. The younger generation is unlikely to forgo a lifetime of pizza and bagels to possibly prevent Alzheimer's seventy years in the future. For persons with vague symptoms such as fatigue, fibromyalgia, rashes, and allergies I would recommend a three-month trial to see if it helps.

THE MEDITERRANEAN DIET

There are thousands of individuals who have always followed a Mediterranean diet. These subjects have volunteered for decades about the health benefits of their diet, and its effect on the risk of dementia. These indicate their incidence of dementia is lower than persons on a Standard American Diet. The Mediterranean diet does include wheat, but the mainstay foods are olive oil, fish, non-starchy vegetables, and lean meat. The Mediterranean diet does not contain rice, corn, potatoes, oats, barley, and minimal dairy, very small amounts of hard cheese such as Parmesan.

One would think it an easy task to prove whether or not the Mediterranean diet was better than the Standard American Diet for the prevention of Alzheimer's disease. Just round up five hundred people over the age sixty-five from southern Italian fishing villages and compare them to five hundred elders living in the US, and compare the incidence of dementia.

The reason this type of trial would not prove the role of diet in the development of dementia is that there are too many other variables besides diet. For instance, the fishermen and women walk much more and climb up and down the stairs of their seaside village every day. As such, they generally are much thinner and physically fitter than Americans. Italian men tend to smoke more than Americans, and the main alcoholic beverage in southern Italy is red wine, consumed during dinner, while Americans prefer beer and hard liquor. Several studies have shown the benefit of one to two glasses of red wine reduce the frequency of heart disease, increase longevity, and reduce dementia. Social isolation contributes to the disease, and elders in Italy are more likely have large, multi-generational families and be included in family activities their entire lives. Many American elders live alone. These are called confounding factors. Ideally in a study there is only one difference between the two study groups. In studies of real people it is very difficult to have only one variable factor.

Dr. Singh and associates, reviewed the medical literature for studies about the effect of Mediterranean diet and the incidence of Alzheimer's disease.[29] The researchers found five previous studies that lasted at least a year and determined the incidence of dementia. They combined the results, which resulted in a study which included over seven thousand subjects, age sixty-two to eighty years. Follow up ranged from two to eight years. Dr. Singh and Associates developed a numerical system to rate adherence to the Mediterranean diet. Subjects self-reported their diet and received one point each for consumption of vegetables, legumes, fruit, cereal, and fish that were higher than average. Subjects received a point if they ate less meat and dairy products than average. They received another point for a daily intake of olive oil, and one point for mild to moderate intake of alcohol (one to two glass of red wine each day). The patients were then divided into low adherence, 0-3 points, medium adherence, 4-5 points, and high adherence, 6-9 points. The subjects were tested for mild cognitive impairment and Alzheimer's disease at the start and finish of the studies.

Dr. Singh's analysis found that a higher adherence to the Mediterranean diet is associated with a reduced risk of mild cognitive impairment and Alzheimer's. Further, the risk of developing dementia was reduced by 8% for each point in the diet compliance scale. In fact, each one-point increase in the diet adherence score reduced the risk of MCI by eight percent. The medium-adherence group showed a twenty percent reduced risk, and the highest diet adherence scores had a thirty-three percent reduced risk of MCI compared to the lowest dietary scores.

Studies about the development of Alzheimer's are difficult. It can take decades for Alzheimer's to develop and very few studies have the funding to follow groups of people for decades. With time, participants move away and drop out of the study, and the number of remaining subjects may be too low to determine proof. Proof is hard to find. Science generally finds correlations that item A is correlated with action B, but that is not considered proof that A causes B.

The lowest level of proof is a testimonial. This is one person claiming great results from whatever product they are endorsing, or selling. Thus Mary Newport's testimonial of her husband's improvement does not carry much scientific weight because there is only one subject.

CHAPTER SIX

WALKING INTO ASSISTED LIVING

Essentially, every family has told me they will never place their beloved family member in a nursing home. Eventually, about ninety percent did.

FOUR STAGES OF DEMENTIA:

Mild Cognitive Impairment refers to having memory difficulty that does not interfere with daily activities. The patient exhibits memory impairment greater than expected for their age, but this does not qualify as dementia. These patients may still be able to work and function at home. However, sixty-five percent of patients with mild cognitive impairment develop dementia within ten years.

Early dementia patients can generally be managed at home. At first, they may be able to manage on their own with services such as Meals-on-Wheels or a caregiver to assist them with shopping and meals. These patients may have some memory loss, but recognize family and friends, and are able to converse. However, they are generally unable to drive or limit their driving to local trips. They may need help managing their finances. Some need to be escorted on all trips outside the home because they easily become lost.

Adult day health care is often a good solution for these patients, and many families like this option. Similar to daycare for children, the elder is dropped off in the morning and picked up in the evening.

Moderate impairment involves difficulty with activities of daily living. These patients need help with dressing, grooming, and bathing. Generally, the patient can no longer prepare meals or use the microwave. They may need help feeding themselves. At this stage, speech is becoming sparse, but they can still engage in conversation, understand others, and perform some activities on their own.

Severe dementia patients are bedbound, have essentially no memory, are able to speak only a few words, and understand very little speech.

DECISIONS ABOUT ADMISSION TO ASSITED LIVING

In my opinion, the primary reason that families choose to admit their loved one to an assisted living facility is incontinence. It is quite burdensome to manage an elder in diapers, and these patients are usually as oblivious to dirty diapers as are young infants. Some adult children find changing their parent's diapers too embarrassing. An adult child's spouse who is the same sex as the elder may find this chore easier to manage. In any case, you or your family should never feel guilty if you cannot manage to care for your loved one at home.

The second most common cause for entering into an assisted living facility is because the patient needs two people to move them in and out of bed, to the chair, or the toilet. In medical terms, this is called a two-person assist. Generally, there isn't a second healthy adult at home to provide assistance twenty-four/seven. An error can result in a fall, and a fracture.

Caring for the Alzheimer's patient is exhausting, even in families with more than one available caregiver. In general, it takes a minimum of three healthy adults to manage an Alzheimer's patient with moderate to severe disease at home. Patients can become combative, wander, or prone to dangerous activities.

Sun-downing is a behavior common with dementia patients even early in the disease process. I have had a few patients in which sun-downing was among the first symptoms of dementia. Although their comprehension may be fairly intact during the day, come sunset, they become agitated, confused, and disoriented. He or she may tremble with fright, but they cannot tell you what they are afraid of. Some patients develop scary delusions such as seeing an intruder in their room. They have difficulty falling asleep or staying asleep. They make wake up in the middle of the night and wander through the house or go outside. One of my patients wandered into the garage and fell over some equipment, breaking an ankle. When she was found missing in the morning, there was a frightening search before she was discovered in the garage.

After three years with dementia, my mother would refuse to open her mouth to have her teeth brushed. Some become extremely distressed by a shower, crying and screaming, fighting every move. It can take three people to shower these patients.

No matter how bad it gets at home, families are often bitterly divided about placing their loved one in an assisted living facility. One adult child may strongly favor this solution, and the other siblings could be violently against the move. Patients' symptoms also fluctuate, which can make the decision even more difficult.

One week the patient may seem better and more competent, and then the next week show reduced function again. So, the family may think that assisted-living is the best choice one week, and then reverse that decision the next.

FINDING THE BEST CARE WITHIN YOUR FINANCIAL MEANS

Cost is always an issue. Usually, one sibling winds up with a higher burden of care than others. The sibling who lives farthest away is usually the one who demands that the parent stay home. And the sibling who provides the most care presses the hardest for the move to assisted living. There are replays of ancient feuds from sibling rivalry to Mom loved you best or gave more money to one sibling over another. I have seen families fight over their inheritance, the caregiving sibling demanding a greater share of the estate. Often, one sibling feels that he or she has been taken advantage of by other family members and that others refuse to help even a little.

The best solution may be to have an aide come to the house for a set period of time, perhaps four-to-six hours each day. Then the family can complete their own chores and errands and the siblings can split the cost for the aide.

There are different levels of credentials for aides. The lowest and cheapest is a companion who has not had any medical training. They cannot assist a person in using the commode or change diapers. Nurse's aide can perform these activities.

The next higher level of credentialed aide, is the CNA, certified nursing aide, who can assist with bathing, assist with transfers from bed-to-chair-to-toilet, and administer medications.

It is possible to hire a full-time live-in assistant, but this is a very costly option, generally as much or higher than the cost of an assisted living facility.

Another decision is whether or not to obtain an aide from an agency. Agencies are also much more expensive than direct-hire help. But they have advantages such as back-up if the primary aide cannot come due to illness or for some other reason. The agency will send out someone else, generally within two hours. Should you direct-hire a companion such as a neighbor, friend, or relative, there could be a day or more when no help is available.

Sometimes the aide may not even call and the patient is left unattended. This can result in a major family crisis as well as a bad outcome. If he or she lives alone, is your beloved elder able to place a telephone call to you or other relatives if his or her caregiver doesn't show up? Will he or she even remember that a caregiver is supposed to be there? If not, it is probably time for assisted living.

An assisted living facility costs can range from $4,000 a month to much more. The last recession has had an impact on assisted living centers, and facilities which had a waiting list for years now have open beds available As many workers lost their jobs and could not find another, I found more and more of my elderly patients were staying at home being cared for by an unemployed family member. This solution is more economic, but the new caregiver usually has no medical training and was sometimes not capable of properly caring for the elder.

Unfortunately, this included caregivers who had substance abuse issues and/or resented or disliked the elder.

My parents used an agency for several years. The caregivers were usually CNAs and provided excellent care. The aide worked from 8 a.m. to 4 p.m. My brother would get home at 5 p.m., prepare dinner, and be available at night. This system worked very well for about four years. Then we discovered a major problem.

Although my mother did not have sun-downing, she did have both insomnia and arthritis. She began to get up at 2 a.m. and wander through the house. She was very quiet and neither my father or brother would awaken. Usually, she would go to the kitchen, get a glass of water and take an ibuprofen for her pain. After one of these nocturnal episodes, they found her unconscious on the bedroom floor the next morning. Dad called 911. When the paramedics arrived they found about twenty of her pills spilled on the floor in the kitchen and twenty more scattered on the dining table.

Martha Jo had a trip to the emergency room which resulted in a three-day stay in the hospital for multiple-drug overdose. No one knows for sure what combination of drugs she took. At first, her doctor thought it was a suicide attempt, but Mom told him and us that she did not try to kill herself. She said her neck hurt and she was only trying to find and take her pain medications which she could not identify. Before this event, we thought she was managing her medications correctly. That was scarily untrue. When I arrived shortly after the overdose on the first of many emergency flights I would take, I did a pill count and discovered that she had been taking twice as much Klonopin, as well as the pain pill, Ultram, that her doctor had prescribed. She was only taking half of her blood pressure medication. After that episode, we locked up her medication. We bought a pill box with divided spaces for each day's dosage to be administered by my father, and kept the large bottles of all the medications in a locked cabinet.

Martha Jo screamed and wept that we didn't trust her. After crying, she was moaning that the people who loved her are the cruelest. She denied making any errors in taking her meds, and refused to believe we were not her enemies. I still recall this unpleasant scene. She tried to get her way by creating guilt. We were trying to protect her from harm. Now I realize that her dementia had progressed much further than I was aware. This was a shocking awakening about the degree of her disability and her inability to recognize that she had made these medication errors. She repeated this same nasty scene for weeks. She and we were lucky that she survived the medicine overdose.

When Christmas arrived and I came for my usual holiday visit, it did not take long before I realized that her condition was much worse. She refused to get up in the morning and had been spending eighteen hours in bed each day. When I checked on her at noon, and again in the afternoon she was awake in her bed. She would assure me that she was fine. She would drink water and could use the bathroom. Around 5 p.m., she would get up to eat dinner, and then watch television until 11 p.m., and then go back to bed until 5 p.m. the following day. No matter what I tried, she absolutely refused to get up. I also noticed that she had a bad cough which she told me she'd had for a month, saying it was only a cold.

I encouraged her to see her regular physician and refused her demand that I just call in a prescription for cough medicine. I'm very glad I made that decision. Although I had to return to California before her appointment, her physician diagnosed her with multiple pulmonary emboli. After lying in bed so long, she had formed clots in her legs which travelled in the veins to her lungs.

Pulmonary embolus is a life-threatening illness. Mom required daily injections of a blood thinner for several weeks which the CNA could not give. Only an RN could administer an injection of the blood thinner. And the original problem of getting her out of bed in the morning still existed. Finally, Dad had her admitted to assisted living for her wellbeing. Even when the shots of blood thinner were completed, he could no longer cope.

I am reluctant to say it, but I think his love for her had died a decade earlier. He did not divorce her; he knew she would be totally lost without him. My father was a veteran, who always did the right thing. He stayed as her husband when he had come to hate her. My mother never knew the truth. If she did, it would have destroyed her. He was tired of her temper tantrums and throwing things at him. It seemed my Dad was the major recipient of her wrath after I had left. It was my dad's decision, not mine, to make; he couldn't handle her anymore.

My father had a severe fall in 2006 which resulted in three compression fractures in the vertebrae in his back. He was in a nursing home for four months, and never fully recovered from this injury. He needed assistance himself after his fall and was not able to care for my mother. My brother resented his caregiver role. Although he was unemployed for two decades and he was staying at their house rent free, he developed a nasty attitude towards both of our parents, even though they were his sole support. I thought it only fair, he lived with them for free, he hadn't worked for twenty years, and he should contribute to their care. That may have been true. I did not know it at the time, but my parents had become more and more demanding and impatient. My parents' nonstop demands on my brother resulted in loud arguments between the three of them. This situation sometimes resulted in my brother getting in his car and driving off to visit friends. I was in California, six hundred miles away, a single parent of a troubled teenager, trying to run a full-time medical practice with no help for myself. Finally I was forced to switch to a part time job to handle my responsibilities.

My mother's admission to assisted living greatly improved my father's and brother's lives. My brother did visit mom twice a week every week, and their relationship became much closer now that the pressure of her daily care was off of him.

At the same time Alzheimer's tore my family apart, I witnessed the destruction of my ex-husband's family. His mother developed Alzheimer's at age seventy. Phyllis had been an excellent seamstress. I noticed she had replaced a zipper on one of my husband's jackets incorrectly, I knew something was wrong. She had installed it so that it didn't zip at all. Phyllis would never have made that kind of mistake.

She was very independent and would drive to the Bay Area in California to visit her sister, a distance of two hundred miles from her home. However, she began to get lost while driving, and she would wind up one hundred miles away from her goal, with no idea of where she was. She had a series of minor accidents, such as driving into a ditch. I watched with disbelief as her husband and sons refused to take away her keys. It seems his family used the emotional coping mechanism of denial. It seemed as if they felt they had no right to interfere with her life. Her husband never did take away the keys.

After the police in Lodi, a town two hundred miles away picked her up, they said her driver's license had expired. After that event, she convinced a neighbor to drive her to the bus station so she could go to visit her sister. Her husband continued to refuse to do anything about it. Finally, I convinced my husband, her oldest son, to go to the bus station to bring her home. He would not have gone if I had not insisted, and it is impossible to say where she might have wound up if she had got on that bus.

Once when visiting her sister, Phyllis began to urinate on herself. Instead of being appalled, she burst out laughing. Her wandering became severe, but because she was physically strong, she was able to easily walk two miles. She was admitted to a group home, but after three months she became violent.

One evening while waiting for dinner to be served, she punched the person sitting next to her. When a friend came to visit, she spat at the woman and cursed her. My father-in-law had to find another Alzheimer's facility twenty miles away that accepted violent patients. Some dementia patients undergo a complete personality change.

When her sister would come to visit, she stayed at their home. Without his knowledge, she began taking her sister's jewelry. Because Phyllis would never wear it again, the sister decided that she could take it. Eventually my father-in-law realized his wife's jewelry was missing. When, he confronted the sister, he told her he thought it was stealing, as Phyllis was still alive and the jewelry still belonged to her. She refused to return it, and he would not let her stay at his house anymore, which caused yet another rift in the family.

My ex-husband never visited his mother during the two years that she was in assisted living. When she fell and broke her hip, my father-in-law was on a trip to Nevada, and the phone number the hospital had was incorrect. The hospital called my husband to come sign the consent for surgery and meet the orthopedist to discuss her surgery, but he refused.

Three days later, her husband came home to discover a dozen phone messages. My ex did not even call his brother, who also lives in town. This upset his brother, and ultimately damaged their relationship to the point that they no longer speak. He never forgave his brother for abandoning their mother. My ex-husband never told me why he didn't visit, other than that he was too busy.

My mother-in-law was not able to cooperate with physical therapy because of her Alzheimer's disease, and she remained wheelchair-bound for the rest of her life, which was one year. There is a fifty percent death rate within one year of a hip fracture among the elderly, and she was yet another statistic.

After my mother-in-law had been in assisted-living for a year, my father-in-law moved in with a new girlfriend. It turns out this is a much more common activity than generally acknowledged. The surviving spouse as caretaker has severe pressure. Not only is the person they loved changed, their spouse isn't there to care for their emotional, sexual, and domestic needs. The caretakers suffer severe loneliness. In effect they have lost their spouse even though they are still living. It is as if the dementia patient is among the un-dead. The length of time until the release of death can be measured in years and decades, which is a very long time to be alone.

Phyllis was never coming back, and the wife who cooked for, traveled with, and loved him no longer existed.

A decade has passed since my mother-in-law died, and I believe that I need to cut my ex-husband some slack. Years after her death, I discovered that both of his parents had alcohol problems. This may explain the lack of intervention of the family about her dangerous wandering and driving. During our marriage I knew my ex was not emotionally close to his mother. He often was rude to her, belittled her, and never sought her company for a visit. There were allegations of abuse from both of his parents towards him as a boy. If his mother was abusive to Stan during his childhood, it would make sense that he would keep his distance and have conflicting emotions about his mother.

A friend of mine who is a social worker mentioned to me there could be another reason for Stan's refusal to visit his mother. She said that some people are ashamed to see their parent's behavior such as acting like a two-year old. They may find being around a demented parent to be so painful, so embarrassing to themselves, their family, and their parent that the only way they can deal with it is to stay away. This isn't because they are selfish, but because they can't bear it.

The last time I saw my ex-husband was at my son's wedding a year ago. I was behind him as he walked to his seat. His gait was very stiff. He seemed less engaged and did not converse as much as he usually does during the reception dinner. He told me that he had taken early retirement and had stopped skiing, camping, and swimming

Recently, I received disturbing news. My son had visited his father and noticed that Stan would sit with a blank look on his face. This is very worrisome to us.

My son has lost both of his grandmother's to Alzheimer's disease and is undecided about whether or not to be tested.

This walk through the process of Alzheimer's disease has taken me to a new place. The place is called forgiveness. I forgive Stan for his faults. Now I see that some of them may have been the first symptoms of his problems. After I forgave him for his sins, it took even longer to forgive myself.

For years I was very angry at myself, for being such a stupid person who fell for his charm and appearance. I forgive myself. I truly loved him for himself. This error in judgment was based in love, and is not a character flaw. After this walk of thirty years, I finally understand what happened to us and our families. I never would have guessed that Alzheimer's was behind some of the earliest painful actions between Stan and his mother. I will do everything I can to stop this horror from devastating other families.

Why do some families of dementia patients manage to come together and survive the experience while others fall apart? One major reason is how the disease affects the patient. If the patient remains calm and pleasant and doesn't cause much trouble, the amount of stress on the family may be manageable. The difficult patients wind up in assisted living at an earlier stage. Caring for Alzheimer's patients who start arguments, have a severe temper, are violent, and wander off takes a huge toll on the family's time, finances, energy, and emotions. It is often unpleasant, and always stressful. No wonder many family members try to avoid the situation. Dysfunctional families simply cannot weather the stress of a serious disease and break apart, whereas a functional family usually can draw together.

The decision to admit a loved one to assisted living is very difficult. The family feels guilty, exhausted, and often isolated. After several years of dealing with the disease, friends and some family members can lose touch. My mother's admission to assisted living was the result of a life threatening illness. My mother in law's admission was due to her dangerous wandering in the neighborhood and inability of her husband to stop it. Each admission has a different family dynamic and a different reason. Sometimes the main caregiver becomes ill themselves, and sometimes a hospitalization is the precipitating event with transfer to assisted living after the acute cause has been resolved.

Caregiver exhaustion occurs, and results in the not-so-nice term granny dump. Each year, just before Christmas, we see a rise in the elderly being brought to the emergency room. The family may indicate that he or she isn't eating or is weak. However, an examination and tests are normal. When the family is called to take their relative home, they cannot be located. No one answers the phone, and then the on-call doctor has to admit the patient as it is usually late at night and adult protective services can't find placement. A day or two after Christmas, the family finally appears at the hospital to pick up grandma. I understand the need for respite care, but there are other ways to do this than the Grandma dump. I personally encountered the granny dump of one or two patients each holiday season.

Once the family has made the decision to seek assisted living, they need to decide what type of facility they would like and how much they can afford to spend.

WHAT TO LOOK FOR IN ASSISTED LIVING.

The group home is very popular because patients live in a regular house. The number of patients is usually limited to between six and twelve. Many times, group homes are family-run businesses with a married couple and their adult children serving as caretakers. Patients may have their own room or share a bedroom. Many patients and families enjoy the home atmosphere and pets are often welcome.

Patients usually have access to the back yard and patio and can enjoy activities such as gardening, putting a golf ball around the yard, playing board games, and making crafts.

The relaxed atmosphere of the group home allows patients and families to become very close to each other, and many people feel that the group home acts like an extended family situation. Group homes can also be less expensive than the more formal and businesslike atmosphere of a professional assisted living care facility.

Group homes are licensed by the state and have to pass safety inspections, such as grab bars in the shower, wheelchair ramps, smoke alarms, and at least one shower that can accommodate a patient in a wheel chair. Personnel must have an active license for Basic Life Support. Someone must be awake and on duty in the home at all times.

Generally, no RNs are on staff, and the patient must go to the Emergency Room or a physician's office for medical assessment. Some group homes will drive patients to doctor visits, some do not. There is usually an extra charge for transportation to appointments. Some cities offer Handi-Ride to disabled patients, but they charge ten dollars a ride, which is much less than a taxi ride. Dementia patients do not do well riding the bus. They forget where they are going and get off at the wrong location and don't know where they are.

Assisted living facilities are also licensed by the state and have many regulations and inspections. Usually larger and more expensive than group homes, the assisted living facility usually has an RN on duty during the day who can make a nursing assessment and decide whether to call the physician or send patient to the emergency room. The RN can also assess whether a patient needs a medicine such as a narcotic.

Assisted living facilities may care from between twelve to three hundred patients. They often offer many activities both on the premises or local trips in a van. They usually have a handicapped-accessible van to take patients to doctor visits, therapy, and shopping or to local events. Some have a professional chef in charge of the kitchen. These larger facilities can provide a wider choice of menu items rather than one meal for everyone.

Assisted living clients are free to come and go as they please. Many assisted living facilities have a designated section specifically for patients with dementia. This area is separate, and these patients must be escorted to the dining room or have their meals served in their rooms. Depending upon the size of the facility, from six to twenty or more rooms are dedicated to dementia patients.

An Alzheimer's unit will have its own activities. It is often called a memory unit, or a butterfly unit because the clients will fly away if left unattended. The memory unit is a locked area.

An increasing number of assisted living facilities specialize in treating only dementia patients. My mother was in a general assisted living center for a year, and then at Barton House, a dementia-only facility in Scottsdale, Arizona for a year. The difference between these two homes was profound. At the general assisted living center, activities were very limited. Martha Jo and everyone else spent the majority of the day in front of a television. Half of the residents appeared to be asleep all of the time. My mother was extremely bored. Just like a young child, she could not understand the plot of a show but could comprehend only the commercials.

The dementia center was much more hands on. Patients rarely spent much time in front the TV. The staff would give my mother a manicure which she really loved. Female guests would also get facials and makeup which they seemed to enjoy very much.

Group activities were conducted at least three times a week. There was a singer who sang Frank Sinatra songs which my mother greatly enjoyed. One lady came every week with two dogs. The guests loved petting and playing with the dogs.

Every holiday had its own special party, such as St. Patrick's Day with special food and hats. Those who could participated in decorations and party favors.

Most important, my mother felt loved by these dedicated caregivers. My brother and I and father were encouraged to participate. We could come for breakfast, and eat with Mom or just have coffee. My mother loved coffee. Her nickname was the Coffee Queen. Although she had lost so much, there were still things in her life that she enjoyed.

The level of care of the medical staff available at assisted living is an important factor to consider when making the decision. This is especially important with respect to the level of care provided at night.

A medical technician has taken a three-month program at a career college and passed the course. This person can dispense prescribed medicine and take vital signs such as blood pressure, heart rate and temperature.

A CNA is a certified nurse assistant. He or she is licensed to bathe patients, can help them change clothes, change diapers, assist in grooming, and help with eating. In most states, CNA's cannot give injections. Most CNA's can change wound dressings.

A medical assistant has completed a course that is generally about nine months. Most work in a physician's office. Then can administer injections, breathing treatments, and do in-office procedures such as EKG and pulmonary testing. They cannot diagnose or treat any medical condition.

A registered nurse can make a nursing assessment, and can follow written guidelines regarding dispensing medications and treatments.

A physician's assistant generally works with doctors in their office or in the emergency room. They complete a two-year program. PA's can assist the doctor during minor surgery, start intravenous line and evaluate patients. A physician's assistant can make an assessment of a patient, just as a registered nurse does. Physician assistants can also prescribe medications. In most states a physician assistant must have a MD as a supervisor who is available by phone if the PA is unsure of the nature of the diagnosis.

When evaluating an assisted living facility, the presence of an RN during the day makes a huge difference. If a patient falls out of bed, he or she can make an assessment whether or not an injury has occurred. If no RN is available, the patient must be sent to the doctor's office or emergency room, an event that is both time consuming and fatiguing. Some medications are written prn (as needed). Only a RN or higher level caretaker can assess whether the situation exists to administer a drug.

A patient may say, "I have a stomach ache."

Only a RN or PA can check vital signs and examine the abdomen. He or she can decide whether it is constipation and order a laxative, gas and order Pepto-Bismol, or if the problem is more severe call the doctor.

If a patient says, "I am short of breath," the RN can listen to the lungs and order a breathing treatment if necessary. RN's note the presence of bed sores or other developments and independently notify the doctor. Dementia patients themselves often do not notice bed sores, rashes, small cuts, or realize their intake of food and drink is low. An RN can detect these from her monthly assessment, which really improves patient care. Of course, assisted living with an RN on the premises eight hours a day costs more than a facility without one.

Don't be afraid to seek another placement if your family or loved one is not happy. Some families stay at the first facility they choose even though they are not happy with various features. Speak up. Most assisted living managers are willing to work with you. If they are not, it's probably time to look elsewhere.

We knew it was time to find a different assisted living when Martha Jo was so unhappy. When I asked her how she was, she would answer "I wish I were dead." We searched and found Barton House which specialized in dementia care. Martha Jo improved so much from this move.

Location
• How far do you have to travel to visit your loved one?
• How close is the doctor's office or the nearest emergency room?

Medical staff and care
• What level of medical staff care is provided? RN? Med-tech? CNA? What level of care is available at night?
• Does the facility have a house physician that visits at least once a month?
• Are all staff trained in CPR/emergency response?
• Does the facility have the care level that you or your loved one requires?

Physical surroundings
• Is it clean?
• Does it smell fresh?

- Is the staff neat and well-groomed?
- Are the floors and common areas clean?
- Is the furniture in good condition?
- Is the kitchen clean? Look at the floors, the walls, the stoves, and overhead fans.
- Are the air vents throughout the facility clean?
- Fire alarms?
- Sprinkler system?
- Hand rails along the corridors? In the bathrooms?
- Emergency call buttons in the bathrooms?
- Trip hazards such as worn carpets or uneven floors?
- Do the windows open? If so, are there safety screens?

Other residents
- Do the other residents seem well-cared for? Happy?
- Do you see them participating in various activities?
- Talk to the residents and their family members. Ask if they would recommend the facility. Ask what they like and dislike about living there. Most assisted living facilities have a front living room where families wait while their love one gets ready to come out. This is a great opportunity to talk to the families of the other clients.

Online reviews
- Check for online reviews of the facilities you are considering.
- Each state will have public records regarding formal complaints from residents and/or families.

Visiting and continuing follow up
- Be alert to the personal care of your loved one. Is he or she clean? Well-groomed? Are his or her clothes clean and neat? Is his or her room/bathroom clean?
- Look for any unusual bruising. If you see something, ask how it happened.
- Observe your loved one's reaction to the caregivers/staff. Does he or she appear happy and confident? Nervous? Fearful?
- Share a meal and observe the food/dining areas. Clean? Is the

food hot? Cooked well? Flavorful? What kind of menu choices and diet options are available?

If something is not right, tell your loved one's aide. If improvements do not occur, speak to the director of the facility, and then give him or her time to investigate and respond. If your parent's situation does not improve after a week or two at most, then consider contacting a help center such as the National Long-term Care Ombudsman Resource Center through its website http://ltcombudsman.org.

Not all bad outcomes at assisted living are abusive. Not far from my home in California, was an assisted living group home. The back yard was surrounded by a six-foot high chain link fence. One day, a spry, eighty-five-year-old Alzheimer's patient somehow managed to climb up and over the fence. He wandered away and, sadly, died. His body was found about three days later in a forested area. The family sued the assisted living facility, claiming negligence. However, the judge ruled in favor of the assisted living facility, citing that California standards for assisted living accept a six-foot fence as adequate. The important thing to remember is to do your best to fit the facility with the needs of your family member.

Life in assisted living is not without its moments of humor. One day, my mother had eaten her lunch. Every bite. Yet, in one hour she came back to the table and demanded lunch. She denied being full and insisted she needed to be fed. One can rarely convince a dementia patient, so the aide served her a second lunch and she ate all of it as well.

By the time a beloved elder has moderate Alzheimer's disease, conversation can become strained. When asked about her day, she says nothing. The give-and-take of a conversation is lacking. What I found helpful on my visits was to bring a photo album. We had at least ten of them dating back thirty years. I would bring a different album to each visit. Mom usually remembered the photographs and enjoyed seeing the faces of her relatives.

Another activity Martha Jo enjoyed was going for a ride. I would take her to church. She could no longer sit through the entire service, but she enjoyed looking at the familiar stain glass windows. We could manage a short trip to Starbucks, or drive out to one of the local mountains that overlooked the city.

Some people say how much their loved ones like to visit the airport. He or she loves to go out to the observation deck and watch the planes take off and land.

Many of my patients' families would get together and remember which activities their parent enjoyed when they were younger. One of my patient's sons recalled how much his mother liked to fish. She couldn't talk any longer, but she did remember how to fish, and she and her son had a very pleasant afternoon at the river.

Did your loved one like music? Find a concert. Did they golf? Visit their favorite golf course. Or bring a putter and golf balls and go out in the back yard and just putt the balls around. Having AD does not mean there is not still some pleasure left in life.

In general, AD patients find movies and plays to be too long and cannot follow the plot. However, they may like cartoons. Watching cartoons from the 1940's and 50's, where each are less than five minutes, can be really enjoyable. One gentleman at Martha Jo's facility liked the Three Stooges. These films are mostly physical jokes instead of word play, and the silly plot is much easier to follow.

Alzheimer's patients are like two-year-olds. Despite a short attention span. they are capable of feeling joy, laughing, and enjoying ice cream. Events such as baseball games, seeing the circus, or a trip to the zoo or a botanical garden all may be appropriate. There is nothing wrong with attending these events. If the patient becomes bored or starts to wander, it is fine to leave early.

We generally think of Alzheimer's as a deterioration of memory, but Alzheimer's also destroys other areas of the brain. Many patients develop a shuffling walk and need to use a cane or walker. They also seem to move in slow motion and may take a full minute to eat one bite of food. Breakfast can easily take an entire hour to eat. Eventually they may have to be fed, just like a baby. A trip to the rest room may take ten minutes.

END OF LIFE AND DNR DECISION

As Alzheimer's unfolds, even basic reflexes are damaged. New-born babies have a swallowing reflex. This reflex is gradually damaged, and then destroyed by Alzheimer's. At first, the patient begins to choke on solid foods such as meat, and must be given a pureed diet. Eventually, the patient chokes on pureed food as well and must switch to a full liquid diet, such as Ensure or Boost. Eventually, even the swallowing reflex is lost. The food just sits in their mouth until it falls out, or the Ensure just runs out again.

When this happens, we reach another major decision point, whether or not to insert a feeding tube. Many families feel that it would be severely cruel to allow their loved one to starve to death. Others believe this is letting nature take its course, and the use of a feeding tube just prolongs the dying process. Generally, when an Alzheimer's patient can no longer swallow, they also cannot speak, and are mostly bedbound. By this stage, they usually have no memory left. Then the question the family must answer is whether the patient experiences any enjoyment in life or do they just exist as a zombie. If it was you, would you want to continue alive in this condition? Families are often divided by the decision about placing a feeding tube. This is why it is extremely important to address this issue with the patient early in the disease or even before it starts. What does your loved one want?

If the decision is to decline the feeding tube then it is time to contact Hospice. Without a feeding tube, patients become dehydrated within 24 to 48 hours. The patients do not die of starvation; they die of infection caused by dehydration. The most common infections are urinary tract infection or pneumonia. Hospice provides pain and anti-anxiety medications to keep the patient comfortable.

I strongly urge every person over the age of sixty to consider advanced directives while they are still healthy and alert. What measures would you want taken? These are separate decisions. Issue number one, do you want a feeding tube? Second decision is whether or not to allow the administration of intravenous fluids. Third, whether or not to allow the administration of intravenous antibiotics Infusions can be done at home or Assisted Living by either a Home Health agency or by a RN on staff at Assisted Living.

The next decision is whether to allow assisted ventilation, having an endotracheal tube placed in the trachea and having a ventilator blow air in and out of the lungs. Many patients struggle against the machine and try to pull the tube out, which results in the patient being sedated for long periods of time. Patients in the intensive care unit can survive living on a ventilator for months. It is a very unpleasant existence.

The next decision is whether cardioversion is acceptable. During cardio-version, the paddles are placed on the chest to restart the heart. An electrical shock is delivered to the front of the chest, to stop the bad rhythm and store the normal sinus rhythm.

Some of my patients required cardioversion when they were still conscious. One gentleman described it as being kicked in the chest by a Missouri mule! Ouch!!

The last decision is whether to accept cardiopulmonary resuscitation. In CPR, the rescuer presses down hard on the sternum, which compresses the heart which lies directly underneath. The goal is to deliver one hundred compressions a minute. Just imagine being socked in the sternum one hundred times a minute. Also, frail bones may fracture. Twenty ribs are attached to the sternum, and they may break and crunch with each chest compression. One oncologist I worked with during my residency called CPR assault and battery on the dying. If there is any consciousness left, CPR and cardioversion must be excruciating.

What you see on television about the success of CPR is inaccurate. There are dozens of hospital and police shows which show gunshot, car crash, electrocution victims, and other acute causes receiving CPR.

In 1996, a medical study was conducted of the portrayal of CPR on television shows. They viewed all episodes of *ER* and *Chicago Hope* during the 1994-1995 season, and fifty consecutive episodes of *Rescue 911* over a three-month period in 1995.[30] CPR was successful in seventy-five percent of the episodes for short-term survival of one hour, and long-term survival, defined as still alive at discharge from the hospital was sixty-seven percent. Only one long-term survivor was shown to have permanent brain damage.

In truth, less than five percent of elderly victims live long enough to recover and return home. Many of the survivors have significant brain damage from the prolonged lack of circulation, and go to nursing homes for the rest of their lives. Also in reality, seventy-five to ninety-five percent of codes are due to cardiac causes. Of persons older than eighty, the odds of surviving a code by more than seven days are less than one percent.

The importance of telling you this is because patients and their families have an incorrect view that CPR is much more successful than it is. A patient may choose to accept CPR, not realizing the most likely result of surviving is long-term nursing home admission with severe brain injury. These shows never mention how painful the procedure is.

Advance Directives are very important, and must be told to spouses and family members. Generally, the primary care physician should also have the needed forms on file. An even better decision might be to see a lawyer and draft the advanced directives with notarized signatures. Then, give a copy to the primary care physician.

Most hospitals now have their own Advanced Directives form which is filled out upon admission. In many states, another form is used for paramedics, who do not accept any other Do Not Resuscitate forms.

For example, in Arizona, the form for DNR for the paramedics is bright orange. This form requires a recent photo of the patient, the doctor's signature, and the signatures of two witnesses who are not relatives.

In the 2008 presidential election, a vice-presidential candidate spoke against the Affordable Care Act. Specifically mentioned was the presence of death panels who would decide if your grandmother would die.

What was really going on is that under current Medicare codes, Medicare will only pay for the treatment of a medical ailment. It will not pay to discuss advanced directives, insurance forms, or any administrative task. Thus, the patient must pay for these office visits. As a result, many people never discussed their wishes with their physician. Under the new ACA codes, Medicare would pay the physician for an appointment to discuss end of life advanced directives. Some physicians do not charge for a simple signature on a form, and charge various amounts per page for other forms.

Unless a completed advanced directives form is on file, the paramedics and hospital staff must attempt resuscitation by law. Even if a family member is present and asks them to stop, they legally must continue unless the doctor of family can provide them with a properly completed, signed, and notarized DNR form with photos.

CHAPTER SEVEN

Walking Around in Circles

My mother drove everyone crazy. Her favorite activity was calling out, "Help me, help me, help me." She sounded sincere and in trouble and would continue however long it took for someone to arrive.

After the nurse or myself came running to ask, "What's wrong Jo?" she would smile sweetly and reply, "Nothing." Then a few minutes later, she would do the same thing again, continuing to say, "Help me," until she received attention. This happened dozens of times each day.

Worse than a two-year-old, she constantly demanded attention. Once the staff finally realized the problem, they gave her lots of one-on-one time, such as doing her nails and giving her a facial. They kept her next to the nursing station so each nurse would greet her every five minutes and she was not left alone for very long. This did help to reduce her attention getting behavior somewhat.

This type of behavior is common in dementia patients. Caregivers work hard not to become irritated with the patients. The patients are not deliberately trying to annoy anyone. They do not remember they've done something ten times in ten minutes and they cannot control their behavior.

One of the volunteers decided to draw my mother's portrait. She loved posing for her picture. However, that picture completely creeps me out. She died on December 21, 2011. The portrait was signed on

December 25 intended as a Christmas gift. Whenever I go home, I turn the portrait down, because I don't like to see it because it was dated after she had died and makes me recall all of the bad events of that week.

I found it easier to think of her as "the thing that used to be my mother," but I discovered there was a better way. One of the nurses at her assisted living facility nicknamed her JoJo, which became her new name. It made it easier for me to think of her as two people; the Martha Jo she used to be, and JoJo the two-year old. Just like a toddler she was in diapers, needed to be fed in the morning, could only speak a few words, but could still smile and laugh. She could no longer bathe or dress herself, and refused to brush her teeth. Not only would she not brush her teeth, she wouldn't let the staff brush them either. She would refuse to open her mouth or she would bite down on the toothbrush. Her gums became very irritated and bled. The dentist suggested a water-pic devise that would at least flush food debris off her gums twice a day.

At meals she ate very slowly. The nurse would give her another bite, and she would pack the food in her cheeks like a squirrel. The food would just sit there packed against her teeth for an hour or two. The dentist said that this was a common problem with dementia patients. It took her thirty minutes to eat a small breakfast.

Finally, she began to choke on solid food and was switched to a liquid diet which helped the bleeding gums as well as the choking. Sometimes she could be coaxed into swishing and spitting out mouth wash. We were afraid all of her teeth would rot, as her teeth were decaying at the gum line.

SOLUTIONS TO COMMON BEHAVIORS

Another annoying problem for us and the staff was that she would only eat dessert. Alzheimer's patients do not have an exclusive on this problem. This is common among geriatric patients in general. As people age, their ability to taste salt, bitter, and sour is reduced. Alzheimer's patients in particular lose the ability to sense aromas.

The loss of the sense of smell is a very early sign of Alzheimer's disease. A scent test can be administered by giving the patient a scented patch and asking him or her to identify the aroma.

When people eat, their nose smells the scents from the food. People note their food has no flavor when then have a cold, what is true is their sense of smell is gone, and the food tastes bland. Among the elderly, the only flavor they detect is sweet. Meat, potatoes, rice, and everything else tastes like it is made of cardboard. So, they refuse to eat it. Solutions include sprinkling sweeteners on food such as stevia, seasoning food with hot sauce, or adding jam to various foods, such as rice or potatoes. If the elder is not getting enough calories from their diet, many families add a high protein drink such as Ensure and Boost. These come in several flavors and taste sweet, so even most picky eaters will drink them.

Patients of all ages may have difficulty swallowing pills. One lady in assisted living had to take fifteen pills a day. This stretched out to a forty-five minute ordeal which left nurse and patient exhausted and unhappy. The standard suggestion is to fill a teaspoon with yoghurt or applesauce and coat the pill so it will slide down the esophagus much easier.

Ask the doctor if some medicines can be discontinued, cut in half, or come in a liquid form. More and more medicines come in a patch, which are easier to use but also more expensive.

Another problem that can appear in even the first stages of the disease is a refusal to change clothing and bathe. One explanation may be that the clothes the patient has on are warm, and the clean clothes are cold. Also, Alzheimer's patients have no sense of smell, and cannot discern if they smell bad. The best solution I found places an emphasis on warmth. Buy a space heater and turn it on fifteen minutes before the shower begins. The area the patient changes clothes should be ninety to one hundred degrees. Run the water in the shower until it is hot, and then adjust to a comfortably warm temperature. It is important the patient isn't waiting, naked, until the water becomes hot. Warm the towels in the clothes dryer immediately before the shower begins. Some patients react to bath time as if it were an assault. This may especially occur if the aide is of the opposite sex of the patient. Female patients in particular may believe they are being raped and fight. If the patient is becoming combative about bathing, I recommend that only aides of the same sex be involved in bathing.

For both males and females have them slip on a bath robe, and have a small hand towel to cover their genitals. Do not attempt to wash their face or hair during the shower or bath if this distresses them. Their hair can be washed at a different time in a salon setting in which the head is extended back over a sink. The face is washed separately during daily grooming with a face cloth. Most Alzheimer's patients hate having water from the shower spray onto their face. For the sake of safety patients should use a shower bench or shower chair.

Another bathroom pathology is the failure to recognize themselves in a mirror. A patient may claim there are bad men, or intruders in their bathroom. This is very frightening to them, and causes much distress. Sometimes, it is sometimes necessary to remove mirrors or cover them up. Likewise, the shadow of a branch on their window at night may be interpreted as an intruder, as they scream and cry out. Or a branch may blow against the window and the squeaky noise causes fear. Check out the window from their point of view and remove tree branches if needed.

Alzheimer's patients live in a fantasy world. They have no recollection of the last two, or three, or four decades. They may believe they are thirty years old, the year is 1970, their children are still small and in school. When they see a reflection of a very old man or woman in the mirror, they have no idea they are looking at themselves. He or she expects to see their thirty-year-old face.

"Who is that old woman?" they think. They may mistake their son for the forty-year-old husband, he now resembles. They mistake their children as their own brothers and sisters. Some may jump back and forth between two time periods, such as early adulthood around age twenty-five into another era of age forty. Their fantasies float and mingle from minute to minute.

Early in the disease it is possible to reorient the patient to reality. If they eventually accept the current year and situation, that is great. However, at some point they can no longer accept the present, and remain in fantasyland for the rest of their lives.

That's why it is important to avoid getting into an argument about reality. You must realize they are delusional, which means having fixed, false beliefs. They remember their past, and dismiss anything else. And it is not possible to convince a delusional person that they are delusional. You must agree with them. If she says this food is rotten, agree. Take it away. In fifteen minutes come back with the same dish and she may accept it. The caregivers have a major advantage, they can remember. The elder will forget what happened in less than five minutes and lives only in the immediate present.

In my opinion, therapeutic lying is essential in the management of dementia. The patient may demand to get in the car and visit a deceased friend. Lie. Tell them the car is in the shop and that they will be picked up in an hour. If the patient is told their friend died twenty years ago, they may cry and grieve. The next time the subject comes up they will cry and grieve again. They cannot remember the death. It is really heart-wrenching to watch this fresh grief over and over because reality is gone for these patients and they are forced to endure the same death a dozen times.

If she asks when her deceased husband is going to come home, again, lie. Tell her he stopped by the store and he will be home soon. She is comforted, and will quickly forget her question.

Another behavior that can try your patience is constantly asking the date and time, even though the clock is right in front of them. Some Alzheimer's patients can no longer read an analog clock. One solution is to take the minute hand off the clock because knowing the hour of the day is adequate. Having digital clocks in every room may help. Try not to roll your eyes or get irritated. They can tell from your face that you are becoming angry and have no idea of why. Most families keep a calendar with very large numbers on it with today's date, generally one in every room.

Every nursing home has patients who complain of theft. Dementia patients often enter the wrong room and do not realize it. They may help themselves to any item and take it. They also usually misplace most of their own belongings as well. Accusations of theft usually arise while the patient is still able to be managed at home.

That's why it is very important to put any valuables such as rings and jewelry in a secure place such as a safety deposit box in a bank.

Take a photo of the items inside the safety deposit box. Then if she complains her necklace is missing, you can say, "Here it is in the safety deposit box where you placed it." This may or may not work. If she doesn't buy it, always agree and lie.

"I will look for it now," is a good answer. Leave the room for a few minutes. She should have forgotten about it by the time you return. However, if she is persistent tell her you will go to the bank, and leave the room again for another ten minutes. She should forget.

JoJo never rummaged, but it can be a very difficult behavior to manage. The patient may spend hours rummaging through drawers, the refrigerator, or the freezer. One patient would rummage through the freezer at two a.m. and leave the door open. The morning mess included a giant puddle on the floor and melted ice cream. When asked what she was looking for she may answer, "None of your business," or "I don't know," but keeps rummaging anyway.

Actually, she doesn't know what she is looking for because she can't remember. One solution is to place a candy bar in the drawer. When she finds the candy she takes it and eats it and stops rummaging.

Think about what your mother would want in the freezer? Place an ice cream bar she likes in a clear wrapper so she can see it. It is probable that she cannot read labels anymore. Another suggestion is to put child-proof locks on the refrigerator, freezer, and drawers. The patient may become very angry about the locks.

One of the clients at Mom's assisted living home was a pacer. He must have walked ten miles a day. It was impossible to stop him. Her facility worked out a course for him. The large backyard had a pathway around the outer yard, and John could pace this all day and be completely safe. The facility was shaped in a square and he could walk around the hallways when it was cold or raining. Everyone was introduced to John. Even the most demented of the other clients would just say "Hi John, this is my room," if he happened to walk in and he would resume pacing the halls.

My parents had a party for their sixty-fourth wedding anniversary. Unfortunately, John was found down in the hallway where he paced, and he died just thirty minutes before their party. He had been a well-known electrical engineer.

Some visitors get upset when they see dementia patients holding a doll. In the patients' minds they are thirty years old and this is their baby. For many of these ladies, being a mother was one of the most important aspects of their lives. Holding a doll brings them comfort. She may not realize it is a doll, but anything that brings serenity is good, and agitation is to be avoided.

A heart-wrenching ordeal to witness is when the patient demands to return home. They have no memory of their dangerous actions that brought them to assisted living, and can't comprehend why they may not go home. When the family reminds them of their previous behavior, the patient doesn't believe it. Understand that you cannot reason with Alzheimer's patients. Most patients' families tell the patient that their doctor has decided they need to be at a home just for now until they get stronger. Another excuse that might work is to remind them their spouse/children cannot care for them at home because they have a bad back and can't lift the patient. Another excuse is their caregiver is going to visit relatives tomorrow. She or he may stop making a scene and accept the excuse, which will be forgotten in five minutes.

It is important the entire family stick to the same story. Also the family must get past the guilt trip that is very common in this situation. It would be very confusing to the patient if one family member says that the patient can go home now and the rest of the family says no.

For the first six months Mom was in assisted living, we did not let her visit our home. We were afraid she would be so upset after she arrived home that she would create a scene, weep, and refuse to leave. When my father finally relented and she came for a home visit, she did very well. She was happy to see her familiar home and her belongings. She enjoyed seeing her piano and paintings. She was supposed to stay through lunch and dinner. However, she surprised us. She took a nap at four, and at five, requested to return to assisted living.

The first visit went well, and then she came to visit the house every other week. However, after about two months she reverted to her previous behavior of throwing a plate at my father and screaming at him for disagreeing with her. Unfortunately, that was the last visit.

At the time, my father was ninety-one and becoming frail. He could barely take care of himself much less deal with her issues.

Another common and unpleasant scene with dementia patients is accusations of infidelity. The totally innocent spouse is shocked, hurt, and defensive. It helps to understand how a dementia patient thinks. They see their spouse talking to a receptionist or nurse. She does not know the person is an employee, and decides the only reason her spouse is speaking to her is that they are having an affair. This is absurd, but this is how they think. It is very hard to not take these accusations personally. Say "I love you." Tell her the receptionist is an employee. Do not get angry, it will make her worse. Leave the room if you need to. Have a nurse or family member take the patient and go to a different room and start a new activity. Do not argue or say she is crazy. She is demented and doesn't know what she is doing.

A similar problem is the patient slaps or hits someone. The patient isn't mean, it is not her real personality. A slap or hit is a statement the patient is confused, angry, stressed, or hungry. The caretaker must back off. Whatever activity was happening when the slap occurred needs to stop immediately, and the patient redirected to some other activity. It may take a caregiver huddle to figure out where the slap came from, what was making the patient angry. Is the sound of the TV too loud? Lack of sleep? Often the patient is feeling pressured to do something they don't like. The patient can't use words to explain, just as when small children hit each other. It is often helpful for care-givers to recall managing their young children and how they would manage a similar situation with a two year old.

The declining mind plays tricks on the patients and families. Try to find triggers for annoying behavior. One lady kept asking if the dog had been fed. It turns out she could see the dog's food dish from where she sat in the living room. Every time she looked at the dish it triggered her question. The solution was to move the dog dish else-where. Then the constant questioning ceased.

The staff at Barton House was very experienced with dementia patients, which is why JoJo improved so much during her stay. I know that staff members are less likely to take behaviors personally and re-main unaffected emotionally, while family members get defensive and angry. The staff had already seen just about every disruptive behavior before and could figure out how to manage it. There is an ability to think like a dementia patient who are irrational, delusional, and exist only in the present. The Alzheimer's Association online at ALZ.org has an extensive file about solutions to problem behaviors available 24/7. So if Mom is taking her clothes off in public, and propositioning her nephew you can reach the hotline any time of day or night.

CHAPTER EIGHT

WALKING INTO HOSPICE

Four years of medical school, three years of internal medicine residency, and thirty years of practice could not prepare me for the day I had to call Hospice of the Valley and register my mother. What did I feel? Guilt, horror, anger at God, and emotional collapse. You may feel all of these emotions too or enter a state of shocked emotional blackout.

Hospice is a Medicare paid program available for any patient who has a life expectancy of less than six months. Although there is a common belief that hospice is only for cancer patients, any patient with a diagnosis of six months or less to live is eligible for hospice care. Hospice is not giving up. It is the decision to focus on keeping your loved one as comfortable and pain free as possible instead of focusing on prolonging life.

As already stated, demented patients do not do well in hospitals or emergency rooms. They become extremely confused, restless, do not understand, and they struggle to resist. They pull out IV's and are oblivious to the pool of blood running down their arm. They pull out urinary catheters, run away, and physically fight the nurses and doctors. The overall experience can be extremely traumatic.

Although I have treated thousands of patients over my career, I can still remember the first night I was on call as an intern. A dementia patient had pulled out her feeding tube which was placed into her nostril to her stomach. She was in her bed, both hands restrained and tied down.

"Please, please let me be." she begged me over and over. She began to sob, and repeated "Please don't do it, you are hurting me."

I still remember her tear-stained face, she must have been ninety. I felt terrible, like the worst heel in the world as I replaced the feeding tube despite her pleas. This was not how I envisioned being the courageous doctor helping people get well and save lives.

Dementia patients in the hospital and emergency room can be dangers to themselves and everyone else. I was in the emergency room admitting another patient when I heard shouting coming from the waiting room. This was followed by a huge crashing sound, and then a security alert was called. A dementia patient had thrown a chair across the waiting room because she was tired of waiting. I saw four burly security officers, one on each limb trying to hold her down and not fracture her brittle bones as she struggled and screamed. She weighed less than one hundred pounds.

Many patients and their families are not aware they can tell their doctor to write an order that says do not transfer to hospital for any reason. Families can also refuse their doctor's recommendations to perform uncomfortable procedures. The mindset of the current medical-legal situation in this country is that every abnormality must be worked up. So if a tiny shadow is seen on a chest x-ray the radiologist recommends a CT scan. Then that report may recommend a biopsy of the lung to be sure it is not cancer. If it is cancer they recommend the maximum treatments. These procedures require the patient to hold still for many minutes, follow directions such as hold their breath and endure a painful needle insertion or worse. If you think the elder will not benefit from these additional tests the medical POA has a right to say no. You will have to sign a refusal form to protect the doctor from litigation.

There have been dozens of malpractice claims against physicians for failure to recommend a full work up on an extremely elderly patient. Huge malpractice awards given to victims in their nineties.

My mother developed several cavities because of her refusal to brush her teeth. However, none of them caused her pain, so we elected to not repair them until or unless they began to hurt.

Hospice patients no longer go to the emergency room or the hospital. Should you decide to send your loved one to the hospital anyway, you must call hospice and cancel that service, otherwise Medicare will not pay for either the emergency room visit or a hospital admission.

With hospice, care is maintained either at home or the assisted-living facility, skilled nursing, or an actual hospice building. Most hospice facilities have a very limited number of beds which are generally reserved for patients without family.

After enrolling in hospice, an intake RN will be sent to conduct an assessment of the patient. They will talk to family and the attending physician and decide if the patient's condition is indeed terminal. A hospice RN will visit the patient each month and make a new assessment, which is signed by the attending physician. At each visit the nurse evaluates the patient to see if they have any needs for comfort. Hospice services include providing oxygen, air bed to prevent and treat bed sores, narcotics including intravenous pain meds for patients with severe pain, medications for nausea, anxiety, diarrhea, constipation, rashes and bed sores. Patients are given a box of these medications so they are available at their home or location, so there won't be a long delay to obtain medication. Usually the regular attending physician is willing to continue as their physician in hospice. Occasionally the primary care doctor declines to continue to provide care, in which case the Hospice doctor will assume care,

How can anyone decide if an Alzheimer's patient has only six months to live? Many patients live with the disease for over a decade. As brain function declines, areas not related to memory are affected. Difficulty walking deteriorates to wheel-chair bound, which becomes unable to stand, which necessitates a two-person transfer into bed and for bathing and toilet. Difficulty swallowing declines into weight loss and aspiration pneumonia in which food goes the wrong way, into the lungs instead of the stomach. If the family has decided to not place a feeding tube, the patient is transferred to hospice when he or she can no longer swallow liquids. If the patient has a feeding tube, time for hospice may come when the patient is bed bound, no longer able to speak, or unable to recognize anyone at all.

The question to ask yourself and discuss with your family members is whether or not any quality of life remains for your loved one. Or, is there only suffering? Hopefully this discussion occurred earlier so family members know what the patient wants.

All hospice patients are Do Not Resuscitate. Entering hospice care requires paperwork, and several forms to complete. One is designating a mortuary and disposition—funeral, cremation, and the type of service.

In general, it is financially better to deal with funeral decisions before the loved ones passes. The emotional shock of losing a loved one, even if their death was expected can cloud your judgment. When you are grieving, it is almost impossible to think straight about these matters such as how much can the family afford for a casket, and whether you want the cost of embalming.

As usual, my parents planned ahead. They both desired cremation, and had purchased a crypt at our church thirty years before they passed. I thank them so much for having these two issues already decided in advance.

You may want to investigate a funeral insurance policy. If your parent or loved one has life insurance, is it enough to cover the cost? If the patient is a military veteran of the United States, you can apply for the VA's death benefit. The benefit is two hundred dollars which is too small an amount for even the smallest funeral. The VA will also provide the flag. You will need the veteran's military serial number and his or her discharge paperwork. Filing this information with Veterans Affairs before a loved one's death is a good idea, as these are just additional chores that have to be done while grieving.

MARTHA JO SUCCUMBS, BUT NOT TO ALZHEIMER'S

My mother had been at Barton House for a year and was doing fairly well. She had finally started to participate in the home's activities and was much happier than in the previous assisted living facility. She had been on the blood thinner Coumadin for two years for treatment of the blood clots in her legs and lungs when she developed a huge bruise on her face. A lab test revealed that her blood was too thin. Her doctor ordered the Coumadin to be withheld for one week, and her blood was to be retested the following Monday.

On Sunday, Mom had a normal breakfast and lunch. Then she lay down after lunch for a nap and simply never awoke again. Her doctor was fairly sure she had a stroke. I affirmed to the nurse that we agreed to Hospice, don't send her to the hospital She was breathing on her own, her pupils were reactive, but she had no voluntary movements. Four days later she passed in her own bed, in her usual nightgown. She passed very gently, with no pain or discomfort, and with our family there.

The events of those last four days are burned into my brain. It was a typical busy Monday morning in my internal medicine office. I had known for months that any day I was going to get a special call.

Finally, it happened. The main nurse from Barton House was on the phone.

"Shelly, come quick," she said. "Your mother is unresponsive, and is not expected to live more than a day or two. Come now."

I stood in the hall, telephone in hand, with every exam room full of sick patients. It was December 19, 2011. The two weeks between Christmas and New Year's Day are often the busiest time of the year for doctors due to influenza and strep.

The Christmas holiday season is also an especially difficult time to get an airline seat. Phoenix is a hub of a major airline, and the local New Year's football game brings in thousands of extra passengers. I had decided that if I couldn't get airline seats, we would drive the six-hundred forty miles, about eleven hours. I managed to snag the last two available seats for my son and I.

We arrived Tuesday afternoon. Mom was in her bed. Her eyes were closed and her breathing was deep and regular. She seemed to be sound asleep. She lay so still. As I held her hand, I noticed her bright red nail polish. This was not a color she ever wore, but I think she had chosen red for Christmas. A little, white stuffed bear sat next to her—a gift from Santa. There had been a Christmas party the day before she fell ill. She did not want to visit Santa, she had too much pride to accept such childish behavior, but the staff brought her gift to her. There was a huge brightly colored fish on her bed. The nurse said they used it as a bolster to keep her on her side. The dedicated staff turned her every two hours to prevent bed sores. She was on an air mattress for the same.

I touched her forehead, she was burning with fever. I caressed her face. She still wore the bright red lipstick she had from her last day. Her face was as pale as death, with bright red pinched cheeks from the fever.

My son, who was twenty-two at the time, could only manage to stay in the room about five minutes, and then he burst out of the nursing home and ran to the car. He didn't want me to see him cry. I stayed with Mom for a while, and then went to comfort my son.

A large high school is located next door to the nursing home. We walked around the track twice, supporting each other. The next morning, my son said he did not want to see his nana, so I went alone. My brother and father couldn't bear it either. My mother was in the same condition, peaceful, asleep. There was no way to tell how long she would last, it could be days. Yet, one hour after I left to get lunch for the family she stopped breathing and passed.

So many times, I have seen families keep a death vigil. Yet, the death often occurs when the family member leaves briefly. It is almost as if the dying person knows the distress they cause, and wait to leave in quiet.

My father, son, brother, and I had just finished lunch when the phone rang. I instinctively knew it could be only one thing. JoJo had just passed. She simply stopped breathing. My father wept. I had never seen him cry during my life. I drove us back to Barton House to say goodbye to her remains before the hearse arrived. Even though her death was expected and imminent, I felt as if I had been punched in the stomach. My brain went blank and I couldn't manage the most simple thought or action. Like many people I didn't really cry until much later.

With hospice, the nurse on call comes out to declare them dead and notifies the attending physician. The mortuary sends the death certificate to the physician for completion. It was two weeks from the day of her death until the certificate was completed.

When a hospice patient passes at home, do not call 911, call the hospice nurse. He or she knows what to do.

My mother died on December 21. My brother's birthday was that week. We went ahead and ate at his favorite restaurant which we had previously planned. JoJo would want her son to celebrate his special day. Later that week, the minister from my parents' church met with us at my parents' home and we planned her funeral while a tiny, one-foot high Christmas tree twinkled on the table. My dad, who was exhausted, agreed with each of my recommendations regarding the hymns and bible verses.

Christmas Eve, 4 p.m., my son and I drove to the mortuary to pick up my mother's ashes. I had invited him to accompany me on this twenty-mile trip as I needed someone to talk to.

I gritted my teeth as we collected the urn. I felt her ghost in the car. Back at home, I walked through the house, trying to find the perfect place to set her urn until her memorial service, which was to be three weeks later. I chose the top of her beloved piano which had been her favorite piece of furniture. Her mother was a music teacher and had given her the piano as a wedding gift. It was her most prized possession. I placed her remains next to the small bust of Mozart which was also a music box.

Now I have that piano, and when I look at it, I remember her giving me my first piano lessons. The bench is covered with a difficult cross stitch pattern she sewed more than fifty years ago and it looks like new. The music box of Mozart still works. I have a baking pan that was hers and an eggbeater. I think of her every time I use these simple utensils.

I had previously purchased food for a Christmas Eve dinner, and cooking dinner that afternoon kept my mind focused. I'm glad I chose to do so because that was the last Christmas our family would ever spend together.

Christmas Day, I prepared breakfast, but my brother chose to go to a restaurant he often ate at on Sunday mornings.

"Come back," I said. "It's Christmas morning."

But he rushed out the door as if pursued by wolves and didn't return until four hours later. I am still not sure why he ran away. My brother was much closer to Mother than I was. He had visited her at least twice a week for two years and had seen her just two days before her stroke. She had been trying to sing, but had forgotten how. He said she was chirping like a bird, singing only one note.

Our flight left at 4 p.m. on Christmas day so we couldn't stay past lunch. No one had purchased any presents and they weren't missed. My son and I flew back to California; we were such a sad pair, grieving on a plane full of happy faces. Everyone else carried gaily-wrapped presents.

When we arrived home at 6 p.m., I gave my son the single gift I had bought him two weeks before our abrupt departure. I hadn't had time to wrap it. We hugged each other.

I had to work the next day and still don't remember a single patient I saw that day.

Sadly, I had used up all of my vacation days at work and could not attend my mother's memorial service. Later, I found out from a family friend that my brother went to pieces in the months following her death. He dyed his hair green and flirted non-stop with women thirty years younger than himself. He was thrown out of a coffee bar for harassing a female patron and then thrown out of a restaurant for the same behavior.

My brother declined over the next few years and ignored his health.

At the end of February, 2012, I decided to not renew my contract at the medical clinic where I worked. My father was ninety-one years old and still living at home, but he clearly could not manage without help. Although his mind seemed intact, he didn't have the emotional or physical strength to keep up with the mail and manage his financial affairs. At Christmas, I had noted massive piles of mail lying around, and his previously clean house was cluttered and dirty.

My father soldiered on, but his health steadily declined. He lost a lot of weight, and was hospitalized twice in 2012. I spent six weeks in Arizona in 2012, and ten weeks in 2013. This decision to retire turned out to be the correct one. During this time, my brother was of minimal help; in fact, his behavior was often part of the problem. My father was supposed to be on a low-salt diet, but my brother would bring home an extra-large pepperoni pizza for dinner. One slice of this pizza contained my dad's entire day's allotment of salt. However, my father would demand to eat some because it smelled so good and he had lost most of his self-control by now. His legs swelled so much that fluid seeped through the skin. I made him homemade soup with no added salt, and bought several cans of low salt soup at a local health food store. I wrote out lists of foods Dad was not to eat, but I know he cheated. The swelling receded a great deal, but my brother kept sabotaging Dad's low salt diet.

Sixteen months after my mother passed, her beloved husband followed her into the grave. Their remains are side by side in the crypt at the church where they were members for forty-five years. My brother and I visit every time I am in town. There is a pleasant fountain, and the tall trees whisper with the slightest breeze. Our parents have a great view of Camelback Mountain. If I stand up in front of their crypt I can see the bright green fairways of the Phoenician golf course highlighted against the bare gray desert rocks. The last time I visited, I left a golf ball and tee on the crypt. Although Dad didn't care for golf, I know that Mom would have liked that.

EMOTIONAL HEALING

Three years have now come and gone since her death. I miss her. She has appeared in my dreams many times now, including last night. My brother calls these dreams visitations, but I don't. He said he never dreams of her. The tyranny of time does not exist in dreams. Sometimes I am a child, a teen, an adult. Some dreams are memories of our home long ago, and some are of events that never existed. She varies in age from forty to eighty-six. Maybe having Alzheimer's is like being inside a dream, past and present, real and imagined jumbled together, illogical upon awaking yet seeming so real at the time.

My faith and church had been a major source of comfort and direction my entire life. I was aware bad things happened to good people since I was a teen when a very good friend of mine age seventeen had died during a camping accident. Faith is tested. I had overseen the deaths of hundreds of patients over the years. My mother's death was the most difficult test I endured, and my faith didn't survive this test.

It is true that good can come from tragedy; people can overcome disability. Is there a spiritual dimension present as my brother believes? Or, are all religions based on delusional thinking, an attempt to make sense of the senseless, a desire to explain the unexplainable? Most religions believe that mortals can manipulate the Divine through prayer and intercession, which never works with Alzheimer's disease. However, faith and prayer do provide peace and comfort during these difficult transitions. It took a long time for our family to realize there was nothing further we could do for JoJo. We did take comfort in the counsel of our minister who reassured us that it was time to let her go.

Some people feel anger towards their deceased parent. I know it sounds irrational, but this is an emotion based on feeling abandoned. Starting with the eulogy, many persons idolize the deceased at first. It can take years to realize emotionally that the parent was not perfect, and the child still has resentments over past mistreatments. Mixed feelings are at war within us, and we are also angry that the deceased is not present to yell at. Then guilt starts. How can I admit to being angry at my mother when she was such a saint?

Give yourself as much time as you need to accept that your parent or loved one had both good features and bad. Whether they tried their best or could have done better, they did what they did for their own reasons and only your acceptance and the irrevocable silence of the grave is left.

Feeling grief is a normal experience. Patients ask me what are the signs between natural grief and depression. First, grief is an expected emotion. If a person feels nothing at all that is abnormal and the grief will come back at a later time often multiplied in strength. Grief lasting than three months is a sign that grief may have turned to depression. Significant weight loss, a sensation that all food has no flavor and an inability to smile at anything are also signs. Being unable to move past grief, to resume hobbies and activities, and constant obsession with the deceased are also signs. Excessive blaming of one self, for not providing more care or thinking the death was your fault are also evidence of depression. Of note, natural grief will not respond to antidepressants. It is okay to seek medical attention, spiritual guidance, and counseling about your feelings.

Being a doctor for so many years had engrained within me the reflex of not feeling anything. I started drinking wine to deal with my buried feelings. Fortunately, a wonderful psychologist was able to help me remove the wall I had placed around my emotions and recover. I know I would not have figured this out on my own. In its own way, the writing of this book is therapy, to share what happened to my family, to my patients and their families as well. Physician, know thyself—easier said than done.

CHAPTER NINE

WALKING INTO THE FUTURE

The Alzheimer's Association has a stated goal of finding a disease modifying treatment for the disease by the year 2025. Many patients and their families are interested in working together with clinical research for a cure.

The National Institute of Health is sponsoring at least a dozen on-going clinical trials for patients at higher risk of AD, as well as testing new drugs and treatments for patients who are already diagnosed with mild cognitive impairment or Alzheimer's disease. Patients at high risk are those who are known to test positive for the mutations associated with early onset disease, or those who have a parent with Alzheimer's disease. If you are interested, you can log on to the NIH website, www.nih.gov, for more information and a list of clinical trials in your area.

REVIEW OF CLINICAL TRIALS

Clinical trials are generally held at large research centers in major cities. Essentially, all require patients to be accompanied by a family member, and have access to reliable transportation. Patients enrolled in clinical trials may be required to submit to repeat blood tests, pet scans, and even spinal taps. Before enrolling there is often a battery of tests, which can be time consuming and fatiguing. Patients need to be cooperative and rested as it takes perseverance and stamina to follow up all of the appointments and complete all of the scans and tests. Any patient accepted into a program needs to make a major commitment to complete the study. Studies vary in length from two months to two years or longer.

Essentially all studies involve a placebo group. Half of the participants will receive the new drug or treatment and half will not. Neither the patient, patient's family, nor the doctors and researchers conducting the study know whether or not the patient is receiving a placebo. If anyone knows, it can affect the results of the randomized tests. Clinicians may subconsciously say leading statements and treat the two groups in a different way. Patients and families may decide the patient is getting worse, and stop the drug and drop out of the study, which may severely affect the outcomes of the research. If a patient believes they are receiving the active drug this knowledge may change their comments about the new drug. They may be reluctant to mention side effects. The placebo effect is very strong, if a person believes the medicine is working they may produce the effect themselves. For instance in studies for sleeping and pain pills, the patients on placebo may have significant improvement, almost as much as the test drug.

Even if the patient becomes worse, it does not mean they are on the placebo. First, the patient may be on the real drug, but the drug might not work for this particular patient even though it may help others. Discovering that a drug does not work is just as important as finding one that does. Also some patients believed to have Alzheimer's may have dementia from another cause. In this case, it isn't that the drug doesn't work it doesn't work on this misdiagnosed patient.

I am not now, and have never been involved in clinical or laboratory research. I have always been in the trenches, seeing patients each day in my office or urgent care.

This overview of current ongoing trails is by no means complete, and will have grown by the time this book is published. Although interest in the research of Alzheimer's disease has been slow, now that the actual mechanisms of how this disease works are coming close to being understood, more direct treatments are being developed. When no mechanism was understood, it was not possible to know where to target the disease.

It is exciting to have much more information to build on. Most drugs are developed in the laboratory. They may start on cultures of brain cells derived from mice or rats or monkeys. Then they are tested on lab animals such as rats or mice. Then there are the first limited studies with human patients to be sure the treatments are safe. This is followed by larger studies involving hundreds of patients. If the drug shows some success, even larger studies are completed until the drug is approved by the FDA and is no longer an experimental medication. This process takes years or even decades.

Several current treatments involve using the patient's immune system to stop or reduce the damage from the disease defining amyloid plaques. Researchers are fairly sure that these treatments must begin before the formation of amyloid plaques.[31] Active immunization is similar to most flu vaccines. A critical part of the amyloid plaque is injected into the patient. The patient's immune system forms antibodies. These antibodies attach to the bad actor, beta amyloid 1-42. After being tagged by antibody, the patient's own immune system will attack the pathological proteins, break them up and digest the remains. One of the first studies of a direct vaccine was conducted in 1999. It seemed to be working well in mice that had dementia, and an early trial was used on humans. Unfortunately six percent of the patients developed an inflammation of the brain itself, which is called encephalitis, and the trial was stopped before completion, as the vaccine was considered unsafe. However researchers believed they have solved the problem of the dangerous side effects. The newer generation of vaccines uses only a small portion of beta-amyloid 1-42, to stimulate the immune system, which is free of the toxic reactions of the original vaccine.

In addition to active immunization, researchers have developed passive immunization. Monoclonal antibodies are made in the lab, directed at various components of the amyloid plaque formation proteins. Making the news for several years is the monoclonal antibody Solanezumab, made by the Eli Lilly Company.[32] This combination of antibody and antigen triggers the person's immune system, which attacks and destroys it. This is how the body's immune system works.

Natural antibodies, made by our own white blood cells, attach to foreign proteins such as bacteria, viruses, and parasites. After our antibodies attach to the enemy, our immune system attacks and kills the invaders. In the case of beta-amyloid, it is a natural product of the body, so our immune system will not attack it. Solanezumab is given monthly by intravenous solution. In the summer of 2015 researchers announced their results of a study of 2,052 patients who received infusions of either Solanezumab or placebo once a month for eighty weeks. The drug did not pass muster of statistical proof that it benefited patients. However, there was an improvement seen in patients with mild disease, and was associated with reduced cognitive decline. The Lilly company has not given up on this drug, an additional study is on-going.

A second drug to treat Alzheimer's disease has just completed phase 2 clinical trials is Aducanumab from Biogen Inc.[33] It is also a monoclonal antibody, directed at a different location on the beta amyloid protein. One hundred and sixty-six men and women with early Alzheimer's disease volunteered. The drug was given by iv infusion at two different doses plus one group with placebo for fifty-four weeks. Patients had amyloid pet scan before and after treatment. The study showed there was a significant reduction in the amount of plaque buildup among treated subjects. The higher the dose and patients treated the longest showed more reduction in plaque. The treated subjects had much less decline in cognitive impairment that those on placebo. A new, larger phase 3 study is starting soon.

There are almost a dozen new drugs being developed and in preliminary studies, mostly conducted by the National Institute of Health. Of note, more than one hundred drugs have already been created to treat the disease and found to be ineffective. So, a cure is not just around the corner. Scientists agree that treatment must begin as early as possible in the disease in order to prevent dementia. Once significant brain damage has occurred, it is too late to treat. New treatments are going to be very expensive. thousands and thousands of dollars, and who will pay for it?

Before enrolling in a clinical trial patients need to realize that going to the office for a monthly infusion is uncomfortable, time consuming, and require the patient to be able to lie still during the infusion. If a patient is irritated, impatient, and uncooperative regarding daily grooming or subject to angry outbursts they might not be a good candidate for a clinical research study.

DISCOVERIES ABOUT THE MECHANISMS OF ALZHEIMER'S

One of the newest and most innovative new treatments involves the use of BRICHOS domain proteins to prevent the beta-amyloid from being folded in the wrong areas.[34] As discussed in chapter three, beta-amyloid cleaved in the 1-42 position forms long sticky fibrils that become toxic. When proteins are manufactured inside cells, very large molecules are present in protein factories which ensure the final product is folded into its correct shape. This research is currently at the laboratory level, determining the mechanisms and biochemistry of a possible prevention treatment, which is still many years away.

The Keck School of Medicine at USC announced a new breakthrough treatment. Mice genetically altered to develop dementia were treated with a virus which increased their production of a protein named interleukin-10.[35] This material caused increased beta-amyloid 1-42 accumulation and worsened the memory of these mice. So, interleukin-10 is a bad guy, worsening the disease. In a companion study mice bred to carry genes known to cause dementia were bred to mice that had a deficiency of interleukin-10.[36] These mice had much less amyloid plaques and pathology of dementia. Several studies have shown this interleukin-10 may be implicated in promoting the damage seen in Alzheimer's disease. Hopeful for the future are vaccines or treatments to reduce interleukin-10 in humans.

When I was in medical school during the 1980's, we were told that neurons were not able to replicate by the time an infant is more than three months old. However, that is not correct. Nerve cells in the hippocampus, which is the major memory center of the brain are able to replicate. Studies conducted at UC San Diego injected nerve growth factor into the hippocampus which is located at the base of the brain.[37] This procedure was done in the operating room, the nerve growth factor was injected bilaterally into ten patients after a small burr hole was drilled through the skull. The patients were followed for several years until they died of other causes. There were no major or even minor complications from the surgery, which was well tolerated. The sample size was very small, ten patients, but the patients did not decline as rapidly as untreated patients. This study will be followed by another using more patients, now that Dr. Rafii has shown this invasive procedure is safe and well tolerated. His study also showed the nerve growth factor was incorporated into the nerve cells in the desired location. It certainly takes a courageous and determined patient to undergo brain surgery to work for a cure.

Lastly there is a possible breakthrough linking the mechanism of Alzheimer's with Mad Cow disease.[38] This disease is caused by a mis-folded protein called a prion. It is much smaller than a virus. The mis-folded protein causes other proteins in the brain and nervous tissue to become misshapen as well, spreading throughout the nervous system. In scrapie, the agent is contagious. Originally found in sheep, the prion is found in the spinal cord and brain. Consumption of undercooked nerve tissue transmits the disease. Symptoms are severe loss of balance, loss of coordination, and dementia. People became infected from eating beef which had eaten contaminated feed from sheep. There are possibilities the beta amyloid 1-42 particles act similar to prions, transmitted one nerve to another and via cerebral fluid, spreading damage throughout the brain. There is no sign Alzheimer's disease is contagious one human to another. But this shows a different model for how the damage occurs. This theory has yet to produce any treatments, but provides a new mechanism of the disease which may result in future treatments.

EXERCISE IS THE BEST PROTECTION

The Alzheimer's Association sponsors several walks for the cure throughout the United states. These are fundraisers and well as increasing awareness of the Alzheimer's Association and the disease. However there are several studies which show running, or any other aerobic activity is actually a proven method to reduce the risk of Alzheimer's disease.

A study by Erickson shows that aerobic exercise forty minutes a day, three days a week for a year, reverses age related atrophy of the hippocampus area of the brain.[39] People lose one to two percent of the volume of the hippocampus starting age thirty as a normal part of aging. Yet just walking reversed this age related atrophy. Can anyone imagine how much money people would pay for a pill which could do the same without any side effects or cost? In fact the aerobic walkers didn't just stop the atrophy, their hippocampus enlarged by an average of two percent after one year. Aerobic exercise is defined as a sustained increase in the heart rate to 135% of normal resting. For persons over sixty, this is a heart rate of 120 to 140 beats. Walking a brisk pace of three miles an hour will suffice. So will ball room dancing, swimming, riding a bicycle at ten to twelve miles an hour, and playing group sports such as soccer. Bowling, baseball, golf, if riding on a cart, are not considered sustained exercise and do not qualify as aerobic. Yoga may have benefits in flexibility and strength but doesn't stress the heart at a consistent level long enough to qualify as aerobic.

A study by Dr. Head found that patients who had exercised the most in the previous ten years, equal to thirty minutes of walking five day a week, had decreased accumulation of amyloid in the brain on pet scans compared to sedentary people.[40] His patients, aged forty-five to eighty-eight years old, who were cognitively normal individuals with a parent with Alzheimer's disease reviewed their exercise pattern for the previous ten years. All patients were tested for the presence of APOE ε4 which greatly increases the risk of disease. Patients positive for the gene reduced their risk of disease by forty percent, a huge difference. Exercisers without the bad gene still reduced their risk of disease by forty percent as well.

QUALITY OF SLEEP

In addition to exercise, quality sleep has been found to help prevent MCI and dementia. Patients with sleep apnea, a condition in which people stop breathing for periods of up to a minute, are at a greatly increased risk of MCI. Their odds are almost twice as high of developing MCI as people with normal sleep patterns. The odds of developing dementia were 1.7 times as high for patients with sleep apnea. When the people stop breathing, the oxygen level in the blood goes down. This is bad for both the heart and brain. Patients with sleep apnea have a triple risk of dying of sudden death and heart attack compared to normal control patients.

Quality sleep turns out to have a major influence of the development of dementia. Caregivers of Alzheimer's patients know all too well these patients have sleep difficulties. Many fall asleep for only an hour or two, then remain awake all night, and sleep all day. However, many of these patients and families recall this person has had insomnia for years and even decades. A change in thinking has occurred, maybe the sleep disorders of Alzheimer's patients are not just an effect of the disease, but an actual cause.

Adam Spira and others studied seventy healthy people without dementia age 56 - 91 in Baltimore MD.[41] Patients completed a survey about their sleep habits, number of hours of total sleep, difficulty falling asleep and frequent awakenings in the previous month. The patients had an amyloid pet scan. Persons with the least amount of sleep had higher amounts of amyloid on their scan, and patients with less than six hours had the most. Trouble falling asleep and frequent awakenings did not seem to matter.

So, the next question is what is it about sleep that could cause such a difference? Sharon Ooms took this one step further and measured the amount of beta-amyloid 1-42 in the spinal cerebral fluid every two hours 8pm to 10 am.[42] One half of the patients were allowed to sleep all night, and one half were kept awake all night. Her results show CSF AB 1-42 levels decreased during a night of sleep and stayed the same for those who stayed awake. This suggests the lack of sleep causes the toxic beta-amyloid 1-42 to build up in the brain.

ALZHEIMER'S IS A WORLDWIDE MENACE

As the future approaches one day at a time, a tidal wave of dementia approaches. The past one hundred fifty years have seen a greatly increased life span for the majority of earth's human inhabitants. The elimination of deadly plagues such as small pox, the development of vaccines for the worse killers such as polio, measles, and influenza, and the development of antibiotics for pneumonia, malaria, staph, tuberculosis, and cholera have reduced infant deaths and the death of billions. There is a worldwide baby boom of children born after 1950. With the reduction of infant mortality, the earth's population has increased from two billion to seven billion people. Birth rates did not start to decline until the 1970's when birth control became more widely available and acceptable. The result is a huge generation of baby boomers, no matter what their native land, that is aging, with fewer children and grandchildren to care for them.

The country with the largest Alzheimer's bomb is Peoples Republic of China. Chairman Mao encouraged couples to have at least four children in the 1950's and 1960's. Women who had given birth to four children received a medal as a Mother of the Country. He seemed to be determined to have a million-man army that would keep China safe and show the world China was strong. However China could never increase its GNP and reduce poverty with this huge population gain, as any gains in economic wealth were wiped out by population growth. The Gross National Product is the amount of economic wealth divided by the population. China's denominator kept getting larger and larger. After the death of Chairman Mao, China developed a one child per couple policy from 1980 to 2016. Now a twenty year old couple can find themselves responsible for four parents, eight grandparents and sixteen great-grandparents. Nursing homes are very rare in China. There is no national health insurance. For millennia it is the duty of the oldest son to care for his parents. But, many of those sons have moved to the city for work, and the parents remain in rural areas. What will happen? Probably the elderly will move to the city and move in with their children. But, who will care for them? China has no Medicare or Medicaid programs; families have to pay out of their own pocket for medicine and doctor visits.

Currently, China has more people with Alzheimer's than any other country.[43] In 1990 China had 3.7 million patients with dementia and 9.2 million in 2010. With a population that is currently 1.2 billion souls, even a one-percent rate of dementia, which is about the overall rate in the US and Europe, would be 120 million individuals.

In this country, California, Florida, and New York have had the largest number of immigrants, although other states bear the burden. More and more refugee families arrive in which one or more of the parents have dementia. San Francisco has been host to families from Afghanistan, Vietnam, China, and Mexico. Here in Central California, 30,000 Hmong arrived from Cambodia in the 1970's after the end of the Viet Nam war. Minneapolis has a large immigrant population from Somalia. Many immigrants are illiterate and come from rural areas. Immigrants older than fifty seem to have substantial difficulty learning English. I have had to use translators as young as six to interpret for their grandparents when these folks come to the emergency room and my office. Most distrust American doctors and medical care. There are various traditional healing methods they have tried before their visit, such as cupping. Patients may have large rings on their backs. Cups are heated and applied to the back to draw out the poison, leaving second degree burns. They may arrive with both dementia and severe medical conditions.

I remember being on-call for the local emergency room. An elderly Hmong patient had been sitting in a chair and fell out of it. The patient did not seem to be able to speak and did not respond to interpreted orders. A CT scan of her head revealed a tumor the size of a baseball in her brain. She must have had this benign tumor for over a decade, but the family thought her lack of speech and movement was simply because she was old. The family decided they wanted everything to be done to help their grandmother live as long as possible and did not understand the situation. Finally the neurosurgeon refused to operate as he felt the patient would not survive the surgery. It took at least a week for me to get this patient discharged back to her home. Some cities have social workers available to assist with disabled immigrants, and some cities do not. In general, whenever there is a budget cut it seems that the social workers are the first to get the ax.

I know from all my years in practice the value of social workers of finding a suitable placement for hospital patients who are well enough to be discharged. Social workers can be worth their weight in gold. Many elderly patients stay at acute care hospitals for weeks waiting for placement and the expenses keep climbing. They are well enough to be discharged, but where? Every nursing home is full and have long waiting lists. Every board and care facility is full. Many of our dementia patients are homeless, and California law states they cannot be returned to their homeless camp under a freeway from whence they arrived.

The arrival of demented elderly in the emergency room, either native or foreign born, is a difficulty that hospitals work hard to solve. The patients have minimal understanding of the situation, are frightened, and are totally dependent on family, who may or may not have their best interests in mind. Some major cities have developed programs to contact immigrant communities about health care and care for the demented. At the hospital we can usually call and get a translator. Using family members as translators may create more difficulty than first appears, as they may not understand medical terms and mistranslate. Many immigrant elders have never eaten American food and refuse to eat or cooperate with medical staff.

One appalling situation I encountered was that of an elderly Chinese lady who had cancer. Originally, she was not expected to survive, but she had. In fact, she was slowly getting better. She was living in her own home with a home health aide. The deed to the house was in her name. She also displayed some early dementia symptoms. The family had believed she would die from the cancer and they would inherit the house. The nurse's aide could not figure out why the patient's children were so cold toward her. It became clear the patient was getting better from the good care she received from the aide. However, the family fired the aide, and brought in an incompetent relative to care for the patient. She died a month later, and family inherited the house. No questions were ever asked, and no charges were ever filed. The aide did call adult protective services and local police, but both declined to investigate the matter.

I can go on and on about really bad situations I have witnessed over the last thirty years. Assuming my colleagues have seen the same amount it is truly tragic to become demented in this country and any other country. Both the elderly and the very young are so vulnerable to exploitation by the families who are supposed to care for them. Even with the legal environment provided in the US, Adult Protective Services and Child Protective Services, these tragic cases keep happening. My local newspaper provides a steady supply of exploited elders and children. With a steady increase in the number of elderly, I am not hopeful for safely in the future. A cure would be really useful about now.

CONCLUSION

We have walked from the golf course to the doctor's office, pharmacy, court house, health food store, assisted living, hospice, and into the future. With all things said and done, I am amazed that the most scientifically proven factors in preventing Alzheimer's are the ones people have heard their entire lives.

- Eat your vegetables. Although my mother did not give us this advice, most moms do and they are right.

- Exercise at least thirty minutes five times a week.

- Avoid sugar and large quantities of refined carbohydrates such as bread, pizza, and beer.

- Don't smoke.

- Control high blood pressure, diabetes, and elevated cholesterol levels.

- Get at least seven hours sleep each night.

- Go to bed at a regular time.

- Do not begin an exercise program or make major changes in diet without clearance from your doctor. Do not exceed recommended doses of vitamins or supplements. Ask your physician about any use of supplements or vitamins.

My mother's dementia was not diagnosed until she was over eighty, and I have decided to not be tested for the known Alzheimer's mutations.

However, as a result of writing this book, I'm taking better care of myself. I take Vitamin D 400IU each day and eat fish once a week. I eat more curry. Fortunately, where I live there is a great Indian restaurant nearby. I also take an omega-three capsule several times a week. I keep active with tennis and swimming three days a week. Weather permitting, I walk two miles seven days a week. I sleep like a rock. Unfortunately, I can't do anything about the DDT exposure in the sixties, but I am doing what I can. So should you.

Together, we can support our local communities and Alzheimer's care groups. Let us all sign up to run for the cure. We are walking into our future. Let's make it as healthy as possible.

REFERENCES

1. www.alz.org/alzheimers_disease_know_the_10_signs.asp.

2. Tombaugh, TN. & McIntyre, N. The Mini Mental State Examination: A comprehensive review. *JAGS* 1992; 40: 922-935.

3. Dotson,V. et al. Recurrent depressive symptoms and the incidence of dementia and mild cognitive impairment. *Neurology* 2010; 75: 27-34.

4. Billioti de Gage, S. et al. Benzodiazepine use and risk of Alzheimer's disease: case-control study. *BMJ* 2014; 349: g5205.

5. Richardson, J. et al. Elevated Serum Pesticide Levels and Risk for Alzheimer Disease. *JAMA Neurology* 2014 March; 71(3): 284-290.

6. www.alz.org/facts/overview:asp.

7. Barnes, DE. & Yaffe, K. The Projected Impact of Risk Factor Reduction on Alzheimer's Disease Prevalence. *Lancet Neurology* 2011 September; 10(9): 819-828.

8. Anderson, H. Alzheimer Disease. Historical Background. *Medscape* 2015 Jan; 15:1-16. emedicine.medscape.com/article/1134817-overview.

9. Sharp, E. & Gatz, M. The Relationship between Education and Dementia An Updated Systematic Review. *Alzheimer Disease Assoc Disorders* 2011 Oct; 25(4): 289-304.

10. Sunderland, T. Clock Drawing in Alzheimer's disease: a novel measure of dementia severity. *JAGS* 1989; 37: 725-729.

11. Johnson, K. et al. Appropriate use criteria for amyloid PET: A report of the Amyloid Imaging Task Force, the Society of Nuclear Medicine and Molecular Imaging, and the Alzheimer's Association. *Alzheimers & Dementia* January; 9(1): E1 - E16. published on line January 28, 2013.

12. Kunkle,F. FDA OKs tool for diagnosing dementia. *Fresno Bee* 2015 August 11; 186: 6 A.

13. Landhuis,E. Advance Warning. *Scientific American* 2015 Spring; 24(1): 72.

14. Gray, S., et al. Cumulative Use of Strong Anticholinergic Medications and Incident Dementia. *JAMA Internal Medicine* 2015 March1; 175(3): 401-407.

15. Wang, J. et al. Unintended Effects of Cardiovascular Drugs on the Pathogenesis of Alzheimer's Disease. *PLOS ONE* 2013 June; 8(6): 1-10.

16. Wong, W. et al. Statins in the prevention of dementia and Alzheimer's disease: A meta-analysis of observational studies and an assessment of confounding. *Pharmacoepidemiology and Drug Safety* 2013; 22: 345-358.

17. Henderson, V. Three Midlife Strategies to Prevent Cognitive Impairment Due to Alzheimer's Disease. *Climacteric* 2014 December; 17 (0 2): 38-46.

18. Bazar, Emily. More people face Medi-Cal death bill. *Fresno Bee* 2015 May 19; 186: 1B,4B.

19. Barnard N. et al. Dietary and Lifestyle Guidelines for the Prevention of Alzheimer's Disease. www.pcrm.org *Physicians Committee for Responsible Medicine* July 2013.

20. Dysken, M., et al. Effect of Vitamin E and Memantine on Functional Decline in Alzheimer Disease. *JAMA* 2014 January 1; 311(1): 33-44.

21. Littlejohns, T. et al. Vitamin D and the risk of dementia and Alzheimer disease. *Neurology* 2014 September 2; 83: 920-928.

22. Canevelli, M. et al. Effects of Gingko biloba supplementation in Alzheimer's disease patients receiving cholinesterase inhibitors: Data from the

ICTUS study. *Phytomedicine* 2014; 21: 888-892.

23. DeKosky, S. et al. Gingko biloba for prevention of dementia: a randomized controlled trial. *JAMA* 2008; 300: 2253-2262.

24. Cederholm, T. et al. Omega-3 Fatty Acids in the Prevention of Cognitive Decline in Humans. *Advances in Nutrition* 2013; 4: 672-676.

25. Spagnoli, A. et al. Long-term acetyl-L-carnitine treatment in Alzheimer's disease. *Neurology* 1991 November; 41: 1726-1732.

26. Duke, J. Tumeric, the Queen of COX-2 Inhibitors. *Alternative & Complementary Therapies* 2007; October: 229-234.

27. Newport, M. *Alzheimer's Disease: What if There was a Cure? The Story of Ketones.* Laguna Beach: Basic Health Publications, Inc. 2011.

28. Perlmutter, D. *Grain Brain: The Surprising Truth about Wheat, Carbs and Sugar—Your Brain's Silent Killers.* New York: Little, Brown and Co. 2013.

29. Singh, B. et al. Association of Mediterranean diet with Mild Cognitive Impairment and Alzheimer's disease: A Systematic Review and Meta-Analysis. *Journal of Alzheimer's Disease* 2014 January 1; 39(2): 271-282.

30. Diem, S. et al. Cardiopulmonary Resuscitation on Television-Misinformation. *New England Journal of Medicine* 1996 June; 334: 1578-1582.

31. Lambracht-Washington,D. & Rosenberg, R. Advances in the Development of Vaccines for Alzheimer's Disease. *Discovery Medicine* 2013 May; 15(84): 319-326.

32. https://www.alzinfo.org/articles/solanezumab.

33. https://www.alzinfo.org/articles/diagnosis/experiental-alzheimers-drug-aducanumab.

34. Knight, S. et al. The BRICHOS Domain, Amyloid Fibril Formation, and Their Relationship. *Biochemistry* 2013 October 29; 52(43): 7523-7531.

35. Chakrabarty, P. et al. IL-10 Alters Immunoproteostasis in APP Mice, Increasing Plaque Burden and Worsening Cognitive Behavior. *Neuron* 2015

February 4; 85: 519-533.

36. Guillot-Sestier, M. et al. IL10 Deficiency Rebalances Innate Immunity to Mitigate Alzheimer-Like Pathology. *Neuron* 2015 February 4; 85: 534-548.

37. Rafii, M. et al. A phase 1 study of stereotactic gene delivery of AAV2-NGF for Alzheimer's disease. *Alzheimer's & Dementia* 2014; 10: 571-581.

38. Walker, L. & Jucker, M. Seeds of Dementia. *Scientific American* 2015 Spring; 24(1): 95-99.

39. Erickson, K. et al. Exercise training increases size of hippocampus and improves memory. *Proceedings of the National Academy of Science* 2011 February; 108(7): 3017-3022.

40. Head, D. et al. Exercise engagement as a moderator of APOE effects on amyloid deposition. *Archives of Neurology* 2012 May; 69(5): 636-643.

41. Spira, A. et al. Self-reported Sleep and beta-Amyloid Deposition in Community-Dwelling Older Adults. *JAMA Neurology* 2013 December; 10(12): 1537-1541

42. Ooms, S. et al. Effect of 1 Night of Total Sleep Deprivation on Cerebrospinal Fluid beta-Amyloid 42 in Healthy Middle-Aged Men. A Randomized Clinical Trial. *JAMA Neurology.* 2014; 71(8): 971-977.

43. MacKenzie, D. China's Alzheimer's time bomb revealed. *New Scientist Health* 2013 June. https://newscientist.com/search/?=China%27s+-time+bomb

www.ingramcontent.com/pod-product-compliance
Lightning Source LLC
Chambersburg PA
CBHW071214020426
42333CB00015B/1406